Contents

List of contributors

Lynne Perry
Olive Tree
1 Minster Close
The Spires
Barry
CF63 1FL

Sally Storey
Head of Business Development
Mayday Health Care NHS Trust
Mayday Road
Thornton Health
Surrey
CR7 7YE

Foreword

One of the more significant features of health care development over the past three decades has been the gradual understanding of the central role of support services. Changes in the nature and provision of clinical care, changes in demography, and the increasingly complex character of treatment with greater numbers of skilled individuals involved with each case all pose problems.

Key figures in the support services are the receptionists and secretaries upon whom patients and health workers depend. To help with their development thirty years ago I wrote *The Medical Secretaries Handbook* and succeeding editions of that book marked the evolution in their roles and status as well as the changing systems within which they worked. This new book moves the process on further. It is written now by practitioners and teachers of the two occupations addressed and that itself says much about how matters have changed. Much that is contained within it really needs a wider audience and many other health care workers would benefit greatly from reading the sections on law and ethics, on audit and quality control and on information technology.

This Foreword does not do justice to the hard work and many wise things that Mari Robbins and her contributors have put into the book. It provides essential background reading that will be of interest to new entrants and to those who have been doing the job already. It covers hospital practice, general practice and work in private practice and will, I believe, become a well-thumbed reference book in the work place as well as the standard textbook for students and those just entering the field of work. For those who design and run the various training schemes it will become an essential course book.

Two elements that occupy the central portion of the book are those referring to communication skills and patient care and this illustrates that in the pursuit of efficiency the prime target; helping the patient make sense of complex systems, is never lost sight of. I have no doubt that other editions will be required as further changes occur but I am equally confident that each edition will continue to provide a better understanding of the real function of us all – personal care.

Michael Drury
Belbroughton 1995

Acknowledgements

My acknowledgements and thanks go to: Jackie Coleman, Practice Manager to Dr S Woolf, General Medical Practitioner, Croydon; Margaret Godfrey, Senior Receptionist, Churchill Clinic, London; and Glenda Webster, Practice Manager/Medical Secretary to Dr Anthony Yates, Consultant Rheumatologist, London.

Thanks are due to Elayne Henderson for reviewing the text.

The National Health Service

History

Prior to the National Health Service Act of 1946, health care in the United Kingdom had developed in an *ad hoc* manner.

The medical profession had, since the latter part of the 19th century, gradually acquired social respectability, legal status and economic strength. The concept of public responsibility for the health of individuals can be traced back to 1834 when the Poor Law Amendment Act was passed which established that parish workhouses should provide sick wards where the able-bodied inhabitants could be treated when they became unwell. However, as the health of the community had been severely neglected, it became necessary for the workhouses to admit the sick paupers from the parish to their wards, who, hitherto, had been left to die as they were unable to obtain medical care themselves. By 1848 the demand for institutional care was such that the sick wards of the workhouses had become entirely devoted to sick paupers. The Public Health Act of that year acknowledged for the first time the State's responsibility for institutional care.

The quality of medical care available improved as scientists made important discoveries. Florence Nightingale, in her contribution both to nurse training and hospital planning, revolutionized the standards of institutional care. Largely due to the philanthropy of the well-to-do and the moral obligations of the charitable and religious bodies, the end of the 19th century heralded the opening of many voluntary and private hospitals. Voluntary hospitals were financed through subscriptions and donations, and attracted the services of skilled doctors, some of whom, acting on their social conscience, treated patients often without payment.

The beginning of the 20th century brought about the advent of insurance schemes which enabled individuals to protect themselves against sickness and injuries which might involve them in expensive medical care or affect their capacity to work.

However, despite the progress that was being made, the standard of medical and nursing care emerging throughout the country was inconsistent both in quality and availability.

At the end of the First World War, the first Ministry of Health was established, which together with various reforms provided the stimuli for a nationally organized health service. The Second World War brought about further reforms and the publishing of the Beveridge Report in 1942 with its recommendations that formed the basis for the post-war system of social welfare services, and the provision of a comprehensive system of health care. Sir William Beveridge recommended that the term `comprehensive' meant that medical treatment should be available for every citizen, both in the home and in hospital, and provided by general practitioners, specialist physicians and surgeons, dentists, opticians, nurses and midwives. He also advocated the provision of surgical appliances and rehabilitation services.

Thus the National Health Service (NHS) became effective in 1948, with the aim of improving the health of the people, to provide health care free of charge and, by eradicating disease, to reduce the demand for free health care services. The NHS took over all hospitals, convalescent homes and rehabilitation units, offering consultants contracts as full-time salaried employees. General medical practitioners providing family doctor services were encouraged to sign contracts to provide family practitioners services for patients in their area, and were permitted to remain self-employed but paid by the health service on a fee basis.

Medical services fell into three functional areas:

- those concerned with the sick person in the community
- those concerned with the sick person in an institution
- those concerned with preventive medical services.

They were identified with the following services:

- the general practitioner services
- hospital services
- services provided by the local authority (excluding school health services).

The hospital service was administered by regional hospital boards, under which were absorbed all the public and voluntary hospitals in the country. The national planning of hospital requirements was established.

Teaching hospitals in England and Wales remained relatively independent with their boards of governors who were responsible directly to the

Secretary of State, but they were linked only to the regional hospital boards in that there was one teaching hospital in each region.

General practitioner services were organized through executive councils, who administered the family doctors' contracts, dental, pharmaceutical and ophthalmic services. The local health authorities administered the preventive services, ambulance services, etc.

The main advantage of the NHS was that it had brought together the services which had previously been under the control of independent organizations. However, administration of this tripartite arrangement was far from satisfactory and in an attempt to improve co-ordination of health care between hospital boards, local executive councils, and the type of care provided by local authorities, the 1974 National Health Service Reorganization Act came into force.

The 1974 reorganization

The 1974 reorganization brought about changes (Figure 1.1) in the way the NHS was organized and structured:

- the formation of regional health authorities (RHAs)

- the formation of area health authorities (AHAs) with directly accountable districts

- community health care, which hitherto had been the responsibility of local authorities, moved to the NHS

- executive councils were abolished and replaced by family practitioner committees (FPCs) to administer family practitioner services (general medical, dental and ophthalmic services, and the pharmaceutical services provided by retail pharmacists).

The changes introduced to the NHS the concept of planning and improvement in personnel and manpower controls.

Community health councils

Community health councils (CHCs) were also created with the 1974 reorganization (generally one for each health district), to represent the interests of the people in their community. Their main function is to make constructive criticisms and recommendations to the health authorities on the provision of services in their district. They also advise patients on how they may make complaints about the services.

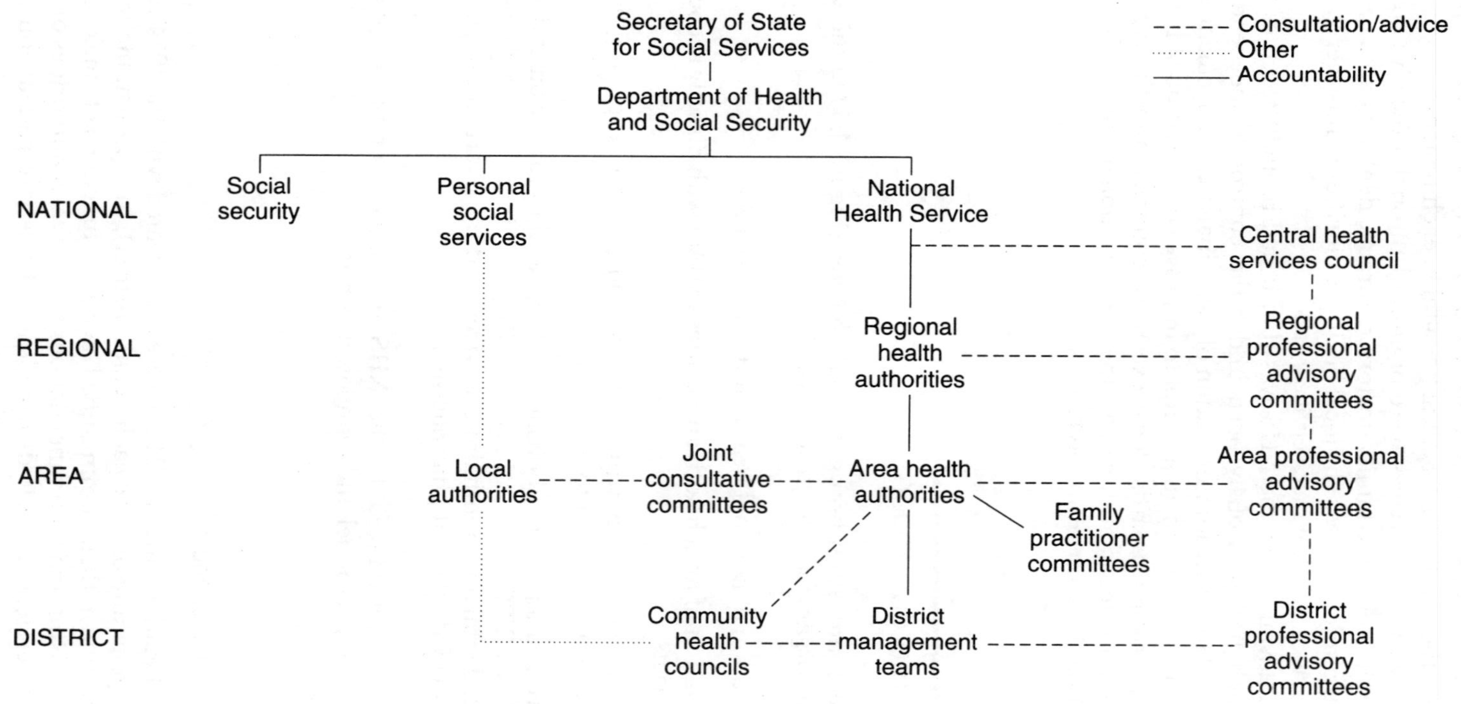

Figure 1.1   The NHS reorganization 1974.

(Source: *Management Arrangements for the Reorganised National Health Service*, HMSO, London, 1972.)

Health service commissioner

Another feature arising from the 1974 reorganization was the appointment of the health service commissioner to investigate complaints within
the NHS, giving complainants direct access to the commissioner. The
commissioner will not investigate a complaint unless he/she is satisfied
that the health authority concerned has had reasonable opportunity to
look into and to reply to the complaint. The commissioner cannot investigate areas covering family practitioner matters. Generally speaking, the
commissioner may investigate complaints in the following categories:

- failure of service
- failure to provide a service
- maladministration.

Regional health authorities (RHAs)

The main responsibilities of the 14 RHAs in England included:

- strategic planning of health services
- capital building programmes
- postgraduate medical, dental and nursing training
- allocation of funds to area health authorities
- appointment of consultants and senior registrars.

The RHA is not involved with the day-to-day running of the health
service.

Area health authorities (AHAs)

Ninety AHAs were set up in England with boundaries in most cases iden-
tical with those of local authorities.
Area health authorities were responsible for planning and providing
services. They determined policies for care provision and put them into
effect with the resources allocated by the regions.

The 1982 reorganization

A major feature of the 1982 reorganization was the elimination of the
middle tier of AHAs, transferring most of the area planning, development

and management functions to DHAs, this gave three planning and management levels in the NHS (Figure 1.2):

- National – the DHSS
- Regional – RHAs
- District – DHAs.

The first aim of this restructuring was one of simplification, and the second to strengthen local level management. These aims were intended to deliver greater efficiency and accountability of the service to Parliament.

FPCs were now directly responsible to the Secretary of State (see Figure 1.2) and were given greater autonomy to manage their own affairs.

District health authorities (DHAs)

The 1982 reorganization divided regions into 192 health districts and for each district a DHA, generally responsible for the day-to-day management

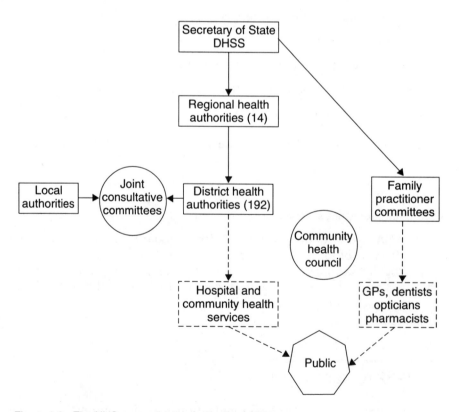

Figure 1.2   The NHS reorganization in England 1984.

of the hospital and community health services and the main functions including:

- day-to-day running of all hospitals
- child health and maternity services
- domiciliary midwifery
- health visiting
- home nursing
- vaccination and immunization
- prevention of disease, e.g. care and after care (health education, chiropody, occupational therapy, etc.)
- school health services (in collaboration with the local education authority)
- health centres
- ambulances.

DHAs which were also the centres for medical teaching had the additional responsibility to appoint consultants and senior registrars.

Organization below district level

Below district level, health services were managed within units, and typically organized on the following basis:

- a large single hospital
- a group of smaller hospitals
- the community services of a district
- client care services, e.g. acute, mental illness or elderly.

Unit general managers were appointed to be responsible for all aspects of the services provided at unit level.

The changing NHS

The NHS in the early 1990s experienced a programme of reforms, more extensive and fundamental than any reorganization since its inception. The changes arose from proposals made in the three White Papers:

- Promoting Better Health – 1987
- Working for Patients – 1989
- Caring for People – 1989.

The Government stated that the proposal for reforms would not affect the basic principles of the NHS to provide a:

comprehensive health service designed to secure improvement in the physical and mental health of the people of England and Wales, and the prevention, diagnosis and treatment of illness.

The reforms required certain statutory changes and these were embodied in the 1990 NHS and Community Care Act.

The most important of these reforms are:

- the introduction of a new system of contractual funding
- measures to manage clinical activity more effectively
- proposals to strengthen management at all levels
- new arrangements for allocating resources.

The NHS reforms and changes were intended to tackle the underlying problems in management and funding of the Health Service. By introducing competition between providers of health services in the form of an 'internal market', the Government intended to increase the efficiency and effectiveness with which resources are used. Services would also be more responsive to users by giving them greater choice. Providers of health services were encouraged to become NHS trusts, taking greater control over the management of their own affairs, including greater freedom to raise capital and to determine staffing structures and rates of pay. The 'purchasers' in this internal market would be either district health authorities (DHAs) or GP fundholders (GPFHs).

The organization of the National Health Service in the early 1990s

The basic structure of the NHS in England following the 1990 reforms is shown in Figure 1.3.

The Secretary of State for Health is responsible to Parliament for the provision of health services. The Secretary of State discharges responsibility through the various health authorities. Community health councils, as

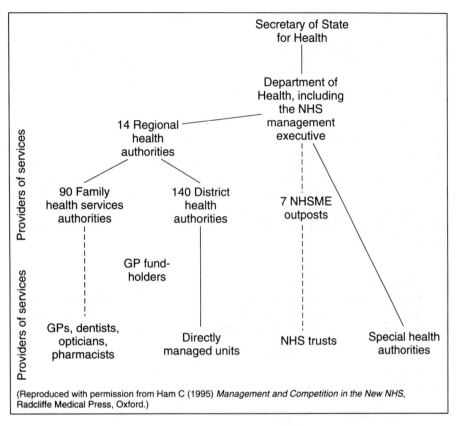

(Reproduced with permission from Ham C (1995) *Management and Competition in the New NHS*, Radcliffe Medical Press, Oxford.)

Figure 1.3   The structure of the NHS in England after 1990.

previously mentioned, are statutory bodies to represent the interests of their local community in the NHS.

As the NHS is almost entirely financed from public funds and with billions of pounds per annum voted to the NHS, Parliament expects some say in how that money is spent.

Department of Health

The responsibilities of the Department of Health cover three areas:

- health
- health care
- social services.

The NHS Management Executive (NHSME) was established in 1991 to have overall responsibility for the management of health services, whilst policy responsibility remained with the Department of Health.

Regional health authorities and NHSME outposts

RHAs were the intermediate tier between the Department of Health on the one hand and DHAs and family health service authorities (FHSAs) on the other. Sub-offices, known as 'outposts' of the NHSME were also set-up to oversee the performance and development of NHS trusts.

District health authorities

Prior to April 1991 DHAs were responsible for managing local health services as well as planning and financing them. With the introduction of the reforms, they became responsible for assessing health needs of their local population, and purchasing hospital and community health services for them. There were 189 DHAs in England, each accountable to their responsible RHA.

Functions of district health authorities:
- Purchasing services for their local community, including services on behalf of non-fundholding general practitioners (GPs), and emergency services for all GPs, including fundholders.

- Managing directly managed units which remained under their control.

- Assessing the population's need for health care.

- Public health.

Family health services authorities

There were 90 FHSAs in England, serving populations ranging from 130 000 to 1 600 000. Each FHSA conformed to a major local authority area and generally followed the geographical boundaries of DHAs.

FHSAs managed the services provided by general medical practitioners (GMPs), general dental practitioners (GDPs), retail pharmacists and opticians. The terms under which family practitioners work are negotiated annually and FHSAs are responsible for implementing the practitioner contracts in their area. GMPs and GDPs are self-employed independent contractors to the NHS.

Functions of family health services authorities:
- Managing the contracts of family practitioners.

- Paying family practitioners in accordance with their contracts and for items of service provided.

- Reimbursement of allowances, etc. to practitioners.

- Planning and developing services to meet those needs.
- Ensuring that quality services are provided efficiently and cost-effectively.
- Carrying out consumer surveys.
- Monitoring medical audit in primary care.
- Monitoring indicative prescribing amounts.

FHSAs were also responsible for:

- approving surgery locations
- checking the standard of surgery premises
- hours of availability of family practitioners
- authorization and monitoring the use of deputizing services.

Special health authorities

Special health authorities administer some NHS services, responsible for specific areas of activity. They are accountable directly to the Secretary of State. Examples include:

- health authorities covering London's postgraduate teaching hospitals
- the Health Education Authority (HEA)
- the Mental Health Act Commission
- the NHS Training Authority (NHSTA).

Community health councils

Community health councils are statutory bodies established by RHAs and continue to represent the interest of the public in local health service provision and act as a channel for consumer concerns. Parliament has agreed that CHCs should have the following rights:

- to relevant information from local NHS authorities
- to access certain NHS premises
- to inclusion in consultation on substantial developments or variations in service
- to send observers to meetings of matching DHAs and FHSAs.

Purchaser/provider split

Since the 1991 reorganization of the NHS, the responsibilities for determining what health care is needed by the population and purchasing accordingly from a range of providers, and those of providing hospital and community health services, have been separated.

Purchasers

- *District health authorities* have relinquished the job of running all hospitals and health units themselves, and buy the services needed by their local population from NHS trusts and other providers, including those in the independent sector.

- *Family health services authorities*, in close liaison with DHAs and local authorities, are also responsible for planning and developing services in primary care in order to meet local health needs.

- *GP fundholders* have their own budget to purchase some 'non-emergency' hospital treatments and community health services for their patients, for example; hip replacement surgery, hernia operations, cataract operations, etc. They can purchase from any provider of their choice. Budgets allocated to GP fundholders are subtracted from those of the DHA.

Providers

Most NHS hospitals and community units are now NHS trusts, providing services to DHAs and other purchasers on a contractual basis.

Services offered by private or independent sector health care providers may be purchased directly by patients through medical insurance, by DHAs or by GPFHs.

NHS trusts can be single hospitals and other health units (mental health services, community health services or services for people with learning difficulties), or a mix of hospitals and health units who have decided to work together, take responsibility for their own affairs and provide services. They are not responsible to RHAs or DHAs, but report to the Department of Health through the NHS Executive.

Contracting in the NHS

Contracts provide the link between the purchaser and the provider. The contracts or service agreements (the Government has stated that such contracts are not legal documents) specify the costs, quality and quantity of care that should be provided.

The following summary will give secretaries and receptionists an understanding of the different types of contract they may come across in their day-to-day work:

- *Block contracts* – A block contract has indicative volumes (usually by specialty) and covers a contract period for a minimum of one year. An annual sum is negotiated prior to the start of the financial year and is paid in 12 equal instalments regardless of variance and activity. More sophisticated block contracts, specifying limits of activity and involving 'triggers' and 'performance payments' in response to variance, now tend to be the most common form of contracting.

- *Cost and volume contracts* – These contracts involve the purchaser paying an agreed price to cover a specified volume of work (a fixed number of episodes for a fixed fee per episode) with agreement being reached prior to the financial year. Each month the provider reports to the purchaser the volume completed, and the purchaser is accordingly invoiced.

- *Cost per case contracts* – These involve a negotiated price for each individual episode of treatment and are normally reserved for special procedures (e.g. cardiac catheterization). They are the usual form of contract with GPFHs.

- *Extra contractual referrals (ECRs)* – These are referrals by a GP not covered by a contract and may be emergencies or 'elective' (those arising from a conscious decision to refer, usually for a condition which is not immediately life-threatening). Emergency ECRs are paid for without question retrospectively, but elective ECRs require prior approval by an officer of the DHA. Both typically occur when a patient needs treatment which is not available from contracted providers, when local waiting lists are considered too long by the GP or when an accident happens away from home.

Combinations or variations of the above contracts may be used to form any other type of contract.

'The Health of the Nation'

The Government's initiative 'The Health of the Nation' published in 1992 is an outline of the intended national health strategy which focuses on health outcomes as well as health care. The approach adopted is:

- select areas for action – or 'key' areas

- set national objectives and targets in key areas
- indicate the action needed by the NHS and other agencies such as local authorities to achieve the targets
- outline initiatives to help implement the action
- set the framework for measuring, monitoring, development and review.

The Health of the Nation initiative initially selected five 'key areas' with nationally determined targets, for example:

- *Coronary heart disease and stroke* – To reduce death rates from both coronary heart disease and stroke to people under 65 by at least 25% by the year 2000.
- *Cancer* – To reduce the death rate for breast cancer in the population invited for screening by at least 25% by the year 2000.
- *Mental illness* – To reduce the overall suicide rate by at least 15% by the year 2000.
- *Sexual health* – To reduce the incidence of gonorrhoea among men and women aged 15 – 64 by at least 20% by 1995, and to reduce the rate of conceptions amongst the under 16 year olds by at least 50% by the year 2000.
- *Accidents* – To reduce the death rate for accidents among children aged under 14 by at least 33% by the year 2055.

Health authorities are encouraged to collaborate and build alliances with local organizations (local authorities, voluntary sector, employers) to achieve the nationally set targets.

The Patient's Charter

Published in 1992, the Patient's Charter is the NHS version of the Government's 'Citizen's Charter' initiative. It emphasizes patient choice and quality of care by setting out national rights and standards. Health authorities are encouraged to add their own local standards, and are held to account by the Department of Health for the publication of local charters and performance against certain standards. The most important of these include:

- maximum waiting times for in-patient treatment and out-patient appointment

- waiting times for assessment and treatment in accident and emergency departments

- numbers of cancelled appointments

- ambulance response times.

The range of standards has been extended from time to time to encompass family doctor services, dental, optical and pharmaceutical services and community care. The Government started to publish 'league tables' of performance in 1995.

Community care

Following the 1990 Act, responsibility for securing care in the community passed to social services departments, together with certain changes in social security payments. This initiative, combined with the Government policy to end long-term institutional NHS provision for people with mental health problems or with learning disabilities, has led to the development of 'joint commissioning' arrangements, whereby health authorities and social services departments work together to secure community care for people in these groups.

Discrepancies in the provision of continuing health care for people with ongoing needs has led to the Government requirement for 'eligibility criteria' to be published by health authorities. These will become effective from April 1996.

Quality of services

An important NHS goal is to improve the quality of services to individual patients, their carers and the wider community. In your own organization you may be part of a team involved in customer-care training, or developing an improved patient complaints procedure.

Audit

Clinical audit is the systematic and critical analysis of the quality of clinical care, including the procedures used for diagnosis, treatment and care, the associated resources, and the resulting outcome and quality of life for the patient (Policy Statement on the Development of Clinical Audit).

Clinical audit embraces the audit activity of all health care professionals, including doctors, nurses and other health care staff. Audit should:

- be professionally led

- be seen as part of an educational process
- form part of routine clinical care
- be based on setting standards
- yield results to help improve outcome of the quality of care
- involve management in the process and outcomes of audit
- be confidential at the individual patient or clinical level
- take into consideration views of the patient and carer
- be an important part of quality programmes.

Secretaries, receptionists and audit

Secretaries and receptionists play an important part in the process of patient care, through their administrative work and their contact with patients. They are often asked to participate in audit activity, for example:

- by recording the times patients arrive at the surgery or clinic, and the actual time they are seen by a doctor
- by attendance at an audit meeting to discuss ways of improving standards.

Remember, the patient's view point and opinion plays an important part in audit, and both secretaries and receptionists are in a good position to hear this view expressed.

Further change: 'managing the new NHS'

Following a review of the 'functions and manpower', the Government published in late 1993 further proposals for change in the organization of the NHS, *Managing the New NHS*. The main thrust of these proposals was threefold:

The 'centre'

Structures were to be simplified and staffing numbers to be reduced in the Department of Health. The renamed 'NHS Executive' (NHSE) would be characterized by more strategic management to ensure accountability, while devolving responsibility to purchasers and providers at a local level. Functions of the NHS Executive would be:

- strategic framework

- policy development for health services

- research and development

- communications

- resource allocation to health authorities

- pay and human resource policy

- performance management and accountability

- public health.

Regional offices of NHSE came into being on 1 April 1994 and would eventually replace both regional health authorities and NHSME Outposts.

Regional health authorities

Legislation was introduced in 1994 to allow the merger of the 14 'old' regions into eight new RHAs:

- North East and Yorkshire

- Trent

- East Anglian and Oxford

- North Thames

- South Thames

- South and West (incorporating the former Wessex)

- West Midlands

- North West (incorporating the former Mersey).

The eight RHAs will be abolished from April 1996. Their functions will be partly devolved to new health authorities and partly taken on by much smaller regional offices staffed by civil servants.

'New' health authorities

During the early 1990s, many DHAs and FHSAs had begun to work closely together to act as health commissioning agencies across primary care and hospital and community health services. One of the main aims was to allow more flexible use of resources in response to trends in medical technology enabling services traditionally provided in hospitals to take place in GP surgeries and public preference for more locally accessible care.

The Health Authorities Act (1995) enabled DHAs and FHSAs to merge formally and this will take effect across the country from April 1996.

A primary care-led NHS

An 'executive letter', *Towards a Primary Care-Led NHS*, issued by the NHSE late in 1994 set out the next phase of the evolution of the Government's health reforms.

GP fundholding expansion

Ministers decided that early experiments in GP fundholding had been successful in improving the quality and efficiency of health care and enhancing patient choice. Therefore, the numbers of GP fundholders would be increased to cover 50% of the population by 1996 and the scope of fundholding would be expanded into three types:

- 'standard' fundholding, covering a wide range of elective procedures in hospital and community services, for practices with a patient list of over 7000
- 'community' fundholding, restricted to the purchase by GPs of community health services only, but enabling much smaller practices to participate in the scheme
- 'total fundholding', whereby practices or groups of practices would take over from the health authority the total budget for all hospital and community health services, including emergency services.

Role of new health authorities

The letter also set out the role expected of new health authorities:

- strategy – developing and implementing strategies for improving the health of the local population, having involved general practitioners in the process

- monitoring – checking the performance and accountability of GP fundholders in securing health services for their patients

- support – providing administrative support and management development to GP fundholders.

The future

In the latter 1990s, the NHS may be entering a period of relative stability and consolidation, although the shift of purchasing power from health authorities to general practice will have very significant implications for the provision of services.

Market competition, envisaged in the White Paper *Working for Patients*, has given way to 'managed competition', where regulatory influences have been re-established to avoid the more traumatic consequences of market forces.

Nevertheless, the NHS continues to face significant challenges which will continue to exert financial pressure on health services. Paramount among these are:

- demography – changes in the age and sex structure of the population which in turn influence the demand for health services (e.g. a greater proportion of elderly people who tend to have greater needs for health care) and the supply of income and labour (fewer people of working age to pay taxes and provide care)

- medical technology – scientific advances tend to mean that more and more health care is possible although often at considerable cost.

These two factors combine to ensure that, as the year 2000 approaches, the ability of the NHS to remain true to its founding principles of comprehensive health care available free to all who need it will be placed under increasing pressure. Many commentators feel that further, perhaps radical, changes to the NHS and the way it is funded and organized may be inevitable.

Summary

The development of the NHS reforms

1988

January	Margaret Thatcher announces Ministerial Review of the NHS.
July	Department of Health created following the splitting up of the Department of Health and Social Security. Kenneth Clarke appointed as Secretary of State for Health.

1989

January	*Working for Patients* published.
November	*NHS and Community Care Bill* published.

1990

June	*NHS and Community Care Bill* receives Royal Assent.
November	William Waldegrave replaces Kenneth Clarke as Secretary of State for Health.

1991

April	NHS reforms come into operation. The first wave of 57 NHS trusts and 306 GP fundholders is established in England.
June	The government agrees guidelines with the medical profession to avoid queue jumping by GP fundholders. A green paper on *The Health of the Nation* is published.

1992

April	The Conservative Party is re-elected. Virginia Bottomley replaces William Waldegrave as Secretary of State for Health. The second wave of 99 NHS trusts and 288 GP fundholders is established in England.
July	A white paper of *The Health of the Nation* is published.
October	The report of the *Tomlinson Inquiry* is published.

1993

February	The government publishes its response to the *Tomlinson Inquiry, Making London Better.* A review of functions and manpower in the NHS is announced.
April	The third wave of 136 NHS trusts and over 600 GP fundholders is established in England.
July	The functions and manpower review reports to ministers.
October	The government publishes its response to the functions and manpower review, *Managing the New NHS.* This includes the proposed abolition of regional health authorities, the merger of district health authorities and family health services authorities, and a streamlining of the NHS management executive.

1994

April   The fourth wave of 140 NHS trusts and 800 GP fundholders is established in England.

October   EL(94)79 *Towards a Primary Care–Led NHS* is published, setting out how GP fundholding is to be expanded and proposing the role of health authorities in future.

1995

April   The 14 regional health authorities merge to become eight.

May   Patient's Charter 'league tables' are published.

July   Stephen Dorrell takes over as Secretary of State.

1996

April   DHAs and FHSAs merge to become 'new' health authorities. GP fundholding is expanded in scope to encompass 'community fundholding' and 'total purchasing'. Eligibility criteria for NHS continuing care became effective. RHAs are abolished.

(Reproduced with permission from Ham C (1995) *Management and Competition in the New NHS*, Radcliffe Medical Press, Oxford.)

2

Patient (customer) care

The medical receptionist and secretary

Medical secretaries and receptionists are important, and sometimes undervalued members of the health care team. Usually they are the first point of contact the patient has with a medical practice or a hospital department, clinic or ward. The receptionist's attitude, empathy and efficiency is able to either enhance or damage its image. A good receptionist can facilitate the way in which a patient accesses the system of medical care and should do all that is possible to make the patient feel welcome, comfortable and to ease the patient's access to medical help and care.

The first impression the patient has of the surgery or hospital department is usually of the reception area and the reception staff. Remember, the receptionist is the 'shop window' and the way in which patients feel as they sit in the waiting area will depend entirely on how the receptionist has reacted and greeted them. It is the receptionist's role to allay patients' fears and worries and help them to feel 'comfortable' whilst they wait. A courteous, friendly manner, accompanied by a smile and an understanding of the situation can work wonders, even with the most difficult of patients. The secretary, too, often has to reassure anxious patients and their relatives, and should adopt a similar approach.

Everyone, whether patients, secretaries, receptionists, doctors or other members of the health care team has feelings. If you have personal problems it is difficult not to allow your emotions to affect the way in which you respond and interact with patients and colleagues. It is important to be aware of this and have the ability to overcome your feelings. Your attitude will influence the attitude of the person you are dealing with. Remember, patients have personal problems too, and are often anxious or frightened, so your empathy of how the patient is feeling will do a lot to improve your own attitude.

How do you welcome patients?

Do you welcome them all in the same way?

Why do you treat people differently?

Why are some patients difficult when attending a hospital or GP surgery?

What are patients' expectations?

Have you experienced feelings of fear?

How do you react when frightened or worried?

How would you like to be treated?

Putting patients first

What is customer care?

Customer care means:

- giving the right impression
- meeting customers' expectations
- exceeding customers' expectations
- listening to customers
- having customer-friendly systems
- being totally professional
- putting customers first
- being totally customer orientated
- having the right attitude
- treating others as you would wish to be treated
- maintaining consistently high standards of service.

Remember the NHS is a very large business organization and the customers are your business

Customer care is not:

- a quick fix
- the flavour of the month
- a campaign which runs for three months, then stops
- just something for the receptionists
- something which brings instant results
- something which starts *after* the patient has reported to the receptionist.

What does the customer expect of us?

Customers have a variety of expectations about:

- the product and service
- staff
- the organization – hospital or GP surgery.

These expectations will include:

- welcoming, pleasant, smiling receptionists
- a concern for their needs
- interest and recognition
- value for money
- adequate information
- good support services
- satisfaction of their needs
- quality service.

Every patient/customer matters and deserves the best you and your practice, hospital or clinic can offer.

Creating the right impression

Some dos and don'ts for creating the right impression

DO	DON'T
Greet the patient pleasantly	Be rude
Make eye contact	
Use names	Be distant, or call everyone 'dear' or 'love'
Give your full attention	Be bored
	Talk to colleagues when patients need attention
Show respect for the patient	Criticize other members of the health care team
Be helpful	Be unco-operative
Say, '<u>May</u> I help you'	Say, '<u>Can</u> I help you'
Be confident	
Be positive	
Be efficient	
Be caring	
SMILE	

What improvements can be made?

By you?

By other members of the team?

YOU NEVER GET A SECOND CHANCE TO MAKE
A FIRST IMPRESSION!

A number of factors help create the right impression, including:

- layout

- space

- signs
- noise
- clutter/rubbish
- staff appearance
- staff behaviour
- facial expression
- tone of voice
- posture.

How to discover the customer's needs

Try to pick up any clues from what is said by the caller, and listen to the 'hidden' message. Do not jump to conclusions about the customer's needs; they are not always clearly expressed.

Follow up and probe by asking questions. Use 'open' questions, starting with:

- How?
- Why?
- What?
- When?

However, do not interrogate the customer.

Actively listen to discover the customer's needs

- Do not make hasty judgements.
- Do not let personal feelings or prejudices prevent you from listening to what is being said.
- Do not interrupt even if you feel you can guess the end of the sentence or remark.
- Do not forget to show that you are listening.
- Do not be distracted.

Body language or non-verbal communication (NVC)

Body language is an important factor in customer care. Remember it may reflect what you are really thinking! Body language should re-enforce the spoken word. When it is contradictory, the customer may well believe the body language and not what is being said.

Important aspects of body language are:

- *Facial expressions and head position* – The face is mobile and can show a huge range of expressions. The expression on your face when you welcome the customer will affect their impression of you. Your head position is also important. Tilting your head to one side indicates interest in the other person.

- *Posture* – The way you hold your body is important. Observe people in your place of work and you will be surprised at the information you can get from their posture. Posture gives an indication of the level of interest in the customer: leaning slightly towards the customer suggests interest and concern; leaning away with arms folded indicates lack of interest or even boredom; standing with hands on hips is an aggressive signal.

- *Proximity* – We all need our 'personal space' – people who get too close to us will often make us feel uncomfortable and threatened. You should be close enough to customers to show interest – approximately three to four feet away is usually the best distance.

- *Eye contact and gaze* – Looking someone in the eye is generally felt to be a positive signal. Look directly at the customer, albeit briefly, when making the initial welcome. Not looking at them may indicate an attitude of not caring. However, some people avoid eye contact for reasons of shyness or of cultural tradition. Your eyes probably give the most expressive signal of all. Watch the customer's eyes during a conversation and you will get feedback of whether they understand/agree with what you are saying. Meet their gaze for approximately two-thirds of the time.

- *Body contact* – In our society it is not correct to touch a complete stranger. Generally the only acceptable form of touching is the handshake when greeting or saying goodbye to a customer.

- *Gestures* – Our gestures give a lot of information, for example, a nod or a shrug. Negative gestures include finger or foot tapping (impatience or aggression) and yawning (boredom).

- *Tone of voice* – We all give a deal of information to people, not by what we are saying, but by the tone of our voice. You may use welcoming words, but if you sound disinterested or angry you may cause the patient distress. Always ensure that your tone is as friendly as the spoken word.

A good technique is to mirror the customer's body language. Customer care and the telephone will be dealt with in Chapter 3.

Complaints within the health service

In recent years there has been increasing public awareness about quality of service. People have higher expectations about the service they receive. It used to be that people only complained if the quality of goods that they bought was shoddy, but nowadays people are equally concerned about how they are treated when buying their goods.

This applies also to the Health Service. People expect to receive a high standard of care and service. If they do not get it they are becoming more vocal about complaining.

Complaints are taken very seriously in the Health Service today. In order to develop and maintain a high standard of service we need to know when things go wrong. We need to know what has happened so that it can be avoided, and that action is taken to prevent it from happening again.

Also, we need to respond to our customers, the patients. If they don't get the service they expect, they need to know that they can complain and that their complaint will be investigated. They need to know that their complaint will be taken seriously and that they will receive an explanation and apology, if appropriate.

Moreover, quality standards are written into the contracts between purchasers and provider units. Complaints as an indicator of quality are monitored scrupulously by the purchasers. If a provider unit's services fall continually below the required standard, it is possible that their contract may not be renewed, thus threatening that hospital's very existence. Also, GP fundholders are unlikely to refer patients to hospitals where there is a high level of complaints about which no action is taken.

Handling complaints – hospital

Your own experience of making complaints should give you an idea of practices which are unhelpful or helpful when dealing with them from the other side of the desk! You will find that most hospitals and medical practices have a standard written procedure for dealing with complaints. If you have not seen one, try to get hold of one.

Complaints procedures

A standard procedure ensures that all complaints are dealt with fairly. Patients will know that they have a right to complain, that their complaint will be taken seriously, and that there will be a thorough investigation. For staff, a standard procedure means that if a complaint is made about them, they will know that it will be investigated fairly.

Having a standard procedure also ensures clear communications. In fact, lack of communication is often the root cause of many complaints made in hospitals. A complaint about a relatively minor matter can become quite serious if it is not handled seriously in the first place. So, having a complaints procedure is better for patients and better for staff (see p. 28). It ensures that complaints are taken seriously, and that everyone involved has an opportunity to express their opinion. It encourages clear communication and by doing so may reduce complaints in the long term. It can help to improve the hospital's public image. More importantly, the major benefit of having a procedure is to ensure that the quality of service can be monitored, thus helping to maintain and develop high standards of care. A standardized procedure makes certain that the charter standard requirement for a full investigation and written response to all complaints from the Chief Executive is met.

Why do people complain?

In hospitals, people complain about a wide variety of different things, for example:

- waiting times (for a first outpatient appointment and in the clinic to see the doctor)
- time on the waiting list
- lack of information
- not being kept informed of treatments
- staff behaviour and attitudes
- food
- cancellation of admission
- cleanliness and building debris
- missing case notes, X-rays and results
- missing property.

Taking customer complaints seriously

All complaints must be taken seriously. If a customer complains, it is an opportunity to put things right.

All complaints should be:

- logged

- passed to the appropriate manager, and

- action taken.

Complaints should be dealt with immediately, and the customer should know the outcome as soon as possible.

Remember, a complaint is any situation where the customer is not satisfied. If a complaint is handled well, the customer might feel more loyalty than before.

Dos and don'ts of complaints

DO	DON'T
Get all the facts	Interrupt
Listen to what the customer has to say	Argue
	Justify
Apologize on behalf of the organization without making excuses	Make excuses
Show concern	
Tell the customer what will be done	

Practice complaints procedure (general practice)

Your practice will have a written protocol of its in-house complaints procedure for the surgery. The procedure details and protocol should be specifically designed and worded to suit the practice. However, it should 'provide an explanation; an apology, if necessary; and indication of action to be taken by the practice to resolve the problem, if that is possible, and to ensure that it does not recur. It should be made clear that the procedure is not intended to apportion blame, to consider the possibility of negligence or to provide compensation' (excerpt from Medical Defence Union Ltd, *Practice Complaints Procedure*).

Remember, a notice or leaflet should be clearly displayed advertising the fact that a practice complaints procedure is available to provide an explanation if concern arises. Figure 2.1 gives an example of a specimen information leaflet.

The majority of complaints arise from failure in communication, either between doctor and patient or receptionist and patient.

Any complaints made directly to staff members should be immediately dealt with according to practice protocol. Remember, sympathy and making time to listen may be all that is necessary to resolve a complaint.

SPECIMEN INFORMATION LEAFLET

(To be given to complainant on receipt of a complaint)

We always try to give you the best services possible, but there may be times when you feel this has not happened. This leaflet explains what to do if you have a complaint about the services we provide for you.

Our practice procedure is not able to deal with questions of legal liability or compensation. We hope you will use it to allow us to look into and, if necessary, put right any problems you have identified or mistakes that have been made.

If you use this procedure it will not affect your right to complain to the family health services authority (FHSA) if you so wish. The appropriate contact addresses for the FHSA and the community health council (CHC) are printed on the reverse of this leaflet. Please note that we have to respect our duty of confidentiality to patients and a patient's consent will be necessary if a complaint is not made by that patient in person.

If you wish to make a complaint, please phone or write to our practice manager. He/she will take full details of your complaint and decide how best to undertake the investigation.

We think it is important to deal with complaints swiftly so you will normally be offered an appointment for a meeting to discuss matters within seven days. Occasionally, if we have to make a lot of enquiries, it might take a little longer, but we will keep you informed. You may bring a friend or relative with you to the meeting.

We will try to address your concerns fully, provide you with an explanation and discuss any action that may be needed. We hope that, at the end of the meeting, you will feel satisfied that we have dealt with the matter thoroughly. However, if this is not possible and you wish to continue with your complaint, we will direct you to the appropriate authorities who will be able to help you.

Figure 2.1   Specimen information leaflet. (Reproduced with permission of Medical Defence Union (1993) *Practice Complaints Procedure*.)

Patients expect:

- an apology, if appropriate
- a clear explanation
- assurance that action will be taken to prevent a recurrence.

Final impressions

The patient must go away feeling satisfied with the level of service you have given. They should feel that you:

- have been willing to help
- have taken a lot of trouble

- are more co-operative than others.

This will give a good impression of:

- you
- your skills as a secretary or receptionist
- your medical practice or your hospital.

Don't take customers (patients) for granted.

Summary

Customer care means that medical secretaries and receptionists should ensure:

- that your customers are, and feel, welcome, e.g. the way you greet them when they arrive will show them how you care
- that you show concern for the customer's needs, e.g. by the way you listen when they are asking a question or explaining something
- that you are interested, friendly and pleasant, e.g. being courteous at all times
- that you know what you are talking about, e.g. the services your hospital, practice or clinic offers
- that the services are the best
- that you recognize each customer as an individual person.

The medical secretary and receptionist and customer care

An experienced receptionist's or secretary's responsibility can be boundless and very fulfilling. They are able to assist and understand patients' medical conditions and help accordingly. They may arrange for a wheelchair, a porter or generally help. They will notice if a patient appears to be distressed and point it out to a nurse or doctor if they think it necessary. On a practical issue, they will keep the reception area generally tidy; magazines will be up to date and in good condition. Toys for children will not become a hazard to waiting patients but kept in a special play area. Plants and flowers will be fresh and watered when necessary. In a private hospital or practice, coffee will no doubt be offered to patients while they wait.

Developing your personal effectiveness

Being assertive

Being assertive means treating other people with respect, asking for what you want and not blaming others for what happens to you. It stems from taking an honest look at strengths and weaknesses and accepting them. Assertive behaviour can include some or many of these mannerisms:

VOICE	steady, firm tone is mid-range, rich and warm sincere, clear
SPEECH PATTERN	fluent emphasizes key words steady, even pace moderate speed
FACIAL EXPRESSION	responsive, matching the feelings expressed open steady features attentive interested
EYE CONTACT	direct maintained
BODY	relaxed open hand movements (inviting to speak) sits upright or relaxed (not cowering or slouching) stands with head held up

This type of behaviour makes other people feel good when they talk to you because you value them and accept their behaviour, and you are not crushed or threatened by rejection because you do not depend on others for approval.

Managing time

To be effective at work good time management is essential. The boxes below identify some of the problems of poor management of time, the causes and some possible solutions.

PROBLEMS	CAUSES	POSSIBLE SOLUTIONS
Having too much to do	Unclear priorities	Check goals or tasks clearly with your manager and check priorities. Each day, decide on your priorities and stick to them
	Wanting to be directly involved with everything	Be selective, delegate if you can
	Unrealistic time estimates	Recognize that everything takes longer than you think – add 20% to your estimates
	Overwhelming pressure and piles of paper	Don't confuse activity with effectiveness – just because you are busy does not mean that you are working well. Try to get into a fixed daily routine with definite times for such jobs as sorting the post, filing, etc.
Inability to finish things	Lack of deadlines	Always set deadlines
	Lack of respect for your time and interruptions by others	Fix a regular time when you need to be left undisturbed. Arrange to divert 'phone calls, and agree to accept colleagues' calls in return. Be sure you know what you want to achieve so that you can communicate this to others
	Doing too many jobs at once	Do one job at a time. When you start a piece of work try to finish it if you can. You waste time each time you have to go back to it, while you remember where you had got to. Be systematic, because if you have to leave a job part finished, it will make it easier for you, or indeed anyone else, to pick it up again
	Wasting time	Handle telephone calls promptly and write messages down immediately. When you make calls, plan what you are going to say beforehand and have all the necessary information to hand

Lack of overview and perspective	Know your priorities. Use your diary. Try to transfer responsibility for some of your work when taking on new jobs. Fix a specific time for any major jobs which should not be interrupted
Laziness	Impose deadlines on yourself and tell others about them

Looking after yourself

There is greater emphasis than ever before on health care staff to work to maintain and improve the health of the community they serve. A variety of initiatives come quickly to mind – antenatal and postnatal care, family planning, child development and immunization clinics, screening (well-man, well-woman, elderly), health promotion programmes for specific conditions (e.g. diabetes, hypertension, asthma), healthy eating and anti-smoking advice, health education literature and posters.

In a more general sense, everyone knows, in theory at least, that they should take certain basic sensible steps to maintain a healthy lifestyle, but for this to become a reality each individual has to understand how they can help themselves to avoid health problems. In doing this, they will also be contributing to their own personal effectiveness at work and at home.

Whether a doctor, receptionist, secretary, or nurse, the message is clear. You will do no one a good service if you do not build in time for looking after yourself.

Paying attention to our own health means taking a hard look at those factors known to contribute to poor health, including smoking, drinking to excess, and being overweight, and making a conscious effort to take exercise, eat healthily, and take advantage of all the health screening checks available.

Handling stress at work

Most people when discussing their jobs would refer somewhere to the amount of pressure they are under at work. Hopefully this will not be a constant problem, and in fact many people claim to work better when under slight pressure. The problems arise when the pressure becomes too great or continues for a long time.

An awareness of the difference between pressure and stress is impor-tant. Generally speaking, stress does not produce a positive or energetic response, but is reflected by panic reactions, irritability, an inability to relax and difficulty with relationships. It is also well known and well established that stress can lead to a variety of medical problems.

Stress at work may have a number of causes. The job may require a great deal of effort, rapid decision making, or its requirements may be ambiguous and therefore leading to competing demands. Unsatisfactory work conditions, inconsiderate bosses or supervisors, shift work and so on can all place pressure on an individual's ability to cope.

Stress is a fact of life and cannot be eliminated. Indeed most people would become quickly bored if too few demands were placed upon them. The key issue, therefore, is that of coping; that is the response made by an individual who encounters a situation with a potentially harmful outcome. Most people use an enormous number of ways of coping with diverse demands, and often different combinations of different types. In general terms there are two major functions of coping. One is to alter the situation causing stress, the other is to deal with the emotion that the stress engenders. The extent to which an individual is able to deal with these two aspects depends on a variety of circumstances. However, the fact that they both have an impact in varying degrees can help in understanding situations better and in developing coping strategies.

Flexibility is important. It is more effective to use a variety of coping skills than one specific response. It is necessary therefore to be cautious when taking on board any fixed ideas on how to cope. However, there are some general guidelines which can help one to think through the situation:

Know yourself and the way you react

Relax

Decide what is important

Look for support from others

Keep communicating

Use a step-by-step, problem solving approach

Patients' rights and National Charter standards

The Patient's Charter, introduced in April 1992, established ten patients' rights and nine specific National Charter standards, which form a central part of the Government's programme to improve and modernize the delivery of the service to the public.

The Patient's Charter

Generally speaking, the Patient's Charter aims to raise the standard of health care provided by the NHS by:

- putting patients' needs first

- providing services that produce evident benefits to people's health

- being an efficient system through better management

- respecting and valuing those who work with and for the NHS.

The National Charter standards are not legal rights as such, but specific standards which the Government looks to the NHS to achieve, as allowed by circumstances and resources.

The standards are:

- *Respect for privacy, dignity and religious and cultural beliefs* – All health services should make provision so that proper personal consideration is shown to the patients, for example by ensuring that privacy, dignity and religious and cultural beliefs are respected. Practical arrangements should include meals to suit all dietary requirements, and private rooms for confidential discussions with relatives.

- *Arrangements to ensure that everyone, including people with special needs, can use services* – All health authorities should ensure the services that they arrange can be used by everyone, including children and people with special needs such as those with physical and mental disabilities; for example, by ensuring that buildings can be used by people in wheelchairs.

- *Information to relatives and friends* – Health authorities should ensure that there are arrangements to inform relatives and friends about the progress of a patient's treatment, according to their wishes.

- *Waiting time for an ambulance service* – When an emergency ambulance is called it should arrive within 14 minutes in an urban area, or 19 minutes in a rural area.

- *Waiting time in outpatient clinics* – A patient should be given a specific appointment time and be seen within 30 minutes of that time.

- *Cancellation of operations* – A patient's operation should not be cancelled on the day he or she is to arrive in hospital. It is acknowledged, however, that this can happen because of emergencies or staff sickness. If, in exceptional circumstances, an operation has to be postponed twice, the patient should be admitted to hospital within one month of the date of the cancelled operation.

- *A named, qualified nurse, midwife or health visitor responsible for each patient* – Each patient should have a named, qualified nurse, midwife or health visitor who will be responsible for their nursing care.

- *Discharge of patients from hospital* – Before a patient is discharged from hospital, a decision should have been made about any continuing health or social care needs that they may have. The hospital has to agree arrangements for meeting these needs with agencies such as community nursing services and local authority social services departments before the patient is discharged. The patient and his or her carers should be consulted and informed at all stages.

Local charter standards

In addition to the stated National Charter standards, the Government requires health authorities to set clear local standards on areas, including:

- waiting times for first outpatient appointments

- waiting times in accident and emergency departments, after the patient's need for treatment has been assessed

- waiting times for taking patients home after treatment where NHS transport is used

- enabling patients and visitors to find their way around hospitals, through enquiry points and better sign posting

- ensuring that staff who deal with patients face-to-face wear name badges.

An extension to the Patient's Charter announced the first national out-patients target:

- Nine out of ten patients referred to hospital by GPs or dentists can expect to be given an appointment within 13 weeks, and everyone can expect to be seen within 26 weeks.

At the same it was announced that:

- The guarantee of a maximum of 18 months' wait for hip, knee and cataract operations is to be extended to cover all admissions to hospital from April 1995.

- In addition, from April 1995, patients can expect treatment within one year for coronary artery bypass grafts and some associated procedures. (If the consultant considers the need for treatment is urgent, patients can expect to be seen more quickly.)

- From April 1995, patients admitted to hospital through an accident and emergency department can expect to be given a bed as soon as possible, and certainly within three to four hours. From April 1996 this standard will be improved to two hours.

The Patient's Charter and the family doctor service

This was published in March 1993 by the Department of Health and the Central Office of Information, and was designed to raise the standards of general practice. However, it sets out the minimum requirements and states that every person in the country has the following rights:

- to be registered with a family doctor

- to change doctor quickly and easily

- to be offered a health check when joining a doctor's list for the first time, or at home yearly, if 75 years old or over

- to receive emergency care at any time through a family doctor

- to have appropriate drugs and medicine prescribed

- to be referred to an acceptable consultant when the family doctor thinks it is necessary, and to be referred for a second opinion if the patient and family think it desirable

- to have access to personal medical records, subject to any limitations by law

- to know that those working for the NHS are under a legal duty to keep the contents of health records confidential

- to choose whether or not to take part in medical research or student training

- to be given detailed information about local family doctor services through the local FHSA directory

- to receive a copy of the doctor's practice leaflet, setting out the services he or she provides

- to receive a full and prompt reply to any complaint made about NHS services.

Access to health care

The first two National Charter standards particularly relate to access to health care for all:

1   Respect of privacy, dignity and religious and cultural beliefs.
2   Arrangements to ensure that everyone, including people with special needs, can use the services.

Consider the ways in which medical secretaries and receptionists ensure that all patients receive the best service and support. This will mean attending to:

- the general needs of all patients and visitors

- the special needs of some patients, especially those of mobility, disability, elderly and ethnic minorities

- patient transport.

Many patients, some of whom will also have special needs, are anxious and uneasy about their visit to the surgery or hospital. The receptionist is usually the first person that a patient will communicate with, and the special skills, knowledge, understanding and empathy that the receptionist uses when receiving and dealing with them are most important.

Patients' general needs

Secretaries and receptionists should be able to answer all queries about the services offered by the practice or hospital department and to direct patients and give appropriate information, for example:

- waiting area
- clinic or surgery times
- relevant consulting room
- toilet, including disabled facilities
- changing facilities
- refreshment facilities (machines, snack bar, etc.).

Patients' special needs

'Disabled' means not being able to do some of the things that able-bodied people can do. A recent survey shows that approximately 15% of adults have some form of disability.

Disabilities may be present from birth, or be the results of accident or disease, which may require a change in lifestyle. However, an ever-increasing group of disabled people are those whose disability comes with age.

The main types of disability are:

- difficulties in mobility

- impaired sight or hearing

- learning difficulties.

People with mobility difficulties may include patients with multiple sclerosis, spina bifida or injury, who are unable to walk and confined to a wheelchair; or the elderly who walk slowly and awkwardly. People with learning difficulties also include those who have difficulty in reading or writing, which still commonly occurs.

Problems may arise when a person with a disability visits the surgery or hospital and may be due to:

- the premises

- the staff

- the patient.

Premises

Look at your place of work in a detached manner and imagine how it must be for a disabled person. Can a patient in a wheelchair readily gain access to the surgery premises or to your hospital department? Are there steps? Are the doors sufficiently wide for wheelchair access? Where can the wheelchair be placed in the waiting area? Is there good light at the reception desk to aid lip-reading? Is there an area or room away from the reception desk where confidential matters may be dealt with, or for a private discussion with a deaf person? Are the notices clearly written and easy to read?

Staff

Empathy is the most important quality for any staff dealing with patients, more so when dealing with disabled patients. Staff should be aware of the disability and anticipate what the difficulties may be, for example, sitting in a waiting room, worrying that a call may be missed makes a deaf person very anxious. Secretaries and receptionists should be tactful and relate to the patient, help with the difficulties caused by the disability and allow more time to deal with their special needs.

Patients

You will find that the majority of patients with a disability are usually less demanding than many other patients. They try to be as independent as possible, although very much aware that special allowances may have to be made because they may be slower, or require things to be written down for them, or, if in a wheelchair, take up more space in the waiting area.

Secretaries and receptionists should be aware that some patients will try to hide their disability, and you should respect their wishes by offering advice without drawing attention to their problems.

Elderly patients

The medical secretary or receptionist should be aware of the many and diverse problems which may affect an elderly patient's access to health care, and try to minimize the effect of some of the following problems which may be encountered:

- impaired hearing
- impaired eyesight
- decreased mobility
- difficulty or inability to cope with new procedures
- reduced energy
- arthritic joints
- fear of being misunderstood
- fear of not understanding instructions
- desire not to be a nuisance to doctors and staff
- socio-economic problems, e.g. financial problems, loneliness, increasing difficulty in day-to-day living.

Cultural issues and language barriers

Medical secretaries and receptionists should be able to identify an individual patient's ethnic or cultural needs and remember that their manner and the way in which they communicate with patients is important in ensuring that ethnic or cultural requirements are identified and met. Remember that, if a patient is discourteous to you, it may be that they have difficulty in expressing themselves or because they are worried about their medical condition. Remain professional, polite and calm at all times.

Interpreters

Good communication plays a vital role in the provision of effective health care. Many patients, especially in inner-city areas, may have a very limited knowledge of the English language and an interpreter may have to be used.

An interpreter may be available in some hospitals, or colleagues within the workforce may be able to help. On the other hand, interpreters are available from external sources and receptionists and secretaries should know how to contact them if it is felt that an interpreter may be of significant help to improve communication and understanding.

Patients may be accompanied by a relative or friend who is more fluent in the English language, when attending surgery or a hospital clinic, to facilitate communication.

Remember that there are still many people in this country who are illiterate. You should be particularly aware and sensitive when offering your help, as they are often extremely embarrassed.

Staff working in general practice will, no doubt, have a list of interpreting services available locally, or will be able to obtain information from their local authority social services department.

The decision as to which is used is dependent upon the purpose for which the interpreter's services are required.

External interpreters should be used:

- for formal communications, for example, interviews, complaints procedures, etc.

- if requested by the patient, relative or fellow professional involved in the care of the patient

- if professional services are deemed to be necessary to enhance understanding.

Visually impaired people

Guidelines are available from the Royal National Institute for the Blind (RNIB) for the provision of a 'user-friendly' environment for people with poor eyesight. These guidelines give suggestions for improving visibility and to providing tactile and auditory clues.

Visibility

Appropriate lighting is the most important aid to vision. People with visual impairment will need twice the quantity of light than sighted people. As people get older, the need for effective lighting increases. The *decor* of the surgery or hospital should reflect the needs of people with impaired sight and the use of contrasting colours will reduce disability. *Shiny surfaces* create reflection and glare; if possible, they should not be used. *Obstructions* must be kept to a minimum and highlighted. Be aware of potential hazards to the visually impaired:

• furniture

• planters

• toys left on the floor.

Ideally, all edges to furniture and walls should be rounded to minimize injury in the event of a collision. *Signs and notices* should be clearly written to be effective.

Any *auditory clues* that may be used must be direct, useful and readily understood.

Tactile clues and texture contrasts can be underfoot, or at a suitable height for hand/finger touch, enabling the visually impaired person to identify a particular area, etc.

All staff who have contact with visually impaired people can do much to facilitate their access to health care.

• Ensure that all instructions are clear and readily understood.

• If necessary take the person to a seat (they may not be able to see it); guide their hand to touch the seat or back of the chair.

• Take them to the doctor's consulting room, or to the nurse.

• Arrange help if they need to go from one hospital department to another.

• Help patients with poor eyesight to fill in forms; if they need to sign their name, place their finger on the place of signature.

• When addressing the patient, use their name, or touch them so they know you are talking to them and not someone else. When you leave them, don't forget to tell them, so that they do not continue a conversation with someone who is not there.

- Use speech appropriate to people with impaired sight.

- Make sure they are sitting safely, and so that the doctor or nurse can see them.

People with hearing difficulties

Patients who have hearing difficulties or who are totally deaf may like to communicate in writing, so make sure you have a supply of pens and paper for this. Perhaps members of staff may be able to use sign language.

If you are dealing with appointments, it is a good idea to make a note in the appointments book of any such patients, so that they are not overlooked when their name is called out and thus miss their appointment.

The following points will help you to communicate effectively with people who have hearing difficulties:

Face-to-face

- Speak up, but do not shout.
- Speak a little more slowly than usual.
- Maintain eye contact.
- Ensure your face is well lit.
- Make sure that the person can see your face clearly to help lip reading.
- Do not look away from the person when talking to them.
- Write it down if you cannot get the message across.

Telephone

- Speak up, but do not shout.
- Speak more slowly than usual.
- If you are not understood, do not repeatedly use the same words, but rephrase what you are saying.
- When giving letters, use letters of the alphabet to clarify ('A' apple, 'C' Charlie, etc.).
- When giving numbers, appointment dates, etc., always ask the person to repeat to ensure understanding.

People with learning difficulties

Staff working in both general practice or hospital will find they are dealing more and more with people with learning difficulties, who are now living in the community, and have the same access to health care as anyone else. It is important that they are treated in precisely the same way, but making allowance where necessary to ensure they get the best out of the health service. Therefore:

- be patient
- do not be intimidated – frustration at not being able to make themselves understood may make them appear aggressive
- stay calm
- ignore any strange mannerisms and comments
- speak in simple, straightforward language.

Remember, there are still patients who are illiterate and experience problems in accessing health care, perhaps when telephoning for an appointment for pathology or ante-natal clinic, for example. Although they may not be able to read what is written down, they may well be able to name individual letters, so be patient and ask them to give you the letters forming the written word, rather than the embarrassment of admitting to you that they are unable to read.

Children

Many children each day attend their doctor's surgery, the local hospital or community clinic. Everything should be done to provide for children's needs, e.g.:

- a play area
- sturdy toys
- colourful books
- a changing area for babies and toddlers.

Again, if possible, chairs and tables in waiting areas should have rounded corners to prevent serious injury.

Children are often frightened by a surgery or hospital, so staff should be sensitive to the special needs of children and do all they can to provide a safe, reassuring and friendly environment.

In 1993 the Audit Commission published a report *Children First* on the care of sick children. The report examined six principles of care and gave guidance as to how each should be adopted:

- *Child and family-centred care* – Hospitals should be sensitive to the special needs of children and their families when in hospital, placing as much emphasis on the care and support of the child (which means the involvement of parents in their care) as on their medical needs. Services also need to be tailored to the wide range of children (from under one up to and including 18 years).

- *Specially skilled staff* – Children should only be cared for by staff specially trained to meet their particular needs.

- *Separate facilities* – Children should only be cared for in facilities which are designed with their needs in mind. Where separate designed facilities do not exist, children should not be treated in other parts of a hospital.

- *Effective treatments* – Children should only receive treatments which are known to be effective.

- *Appropriate hospitalization* – Children should only be admitted to hospital when the treatment and care cannot be provided in an alternative environment, e.g. their home.

- *Strategic commissioning* – Purchasers should be commissioning the types of service which most meets children's needs, particularly the development of hospital-at-home services to avoid hospitalization as far as possible.

- *The National Association for the Welfare of Children in Hospital (NAWCH)* has added to these in its Charter for Children in Hospital.

Working people

General practitioners and hospitals alike are becoming aware of the need to improve access to health care for working men and women by offering appointments at times better suited to their working hours. As a result surgeries and clinics are either offering appointments earlier in the morning, later in the evening, or reserving the first appointments for business people. Similar consideration is being given to mothers with children at school and to the elderly by offering appointments at appropriate times during the day.

Transport

Patients with their own transport

Many patients will attend both hospital and general practice by car and, although hospitals are now providing more car-parking facilities for all patients, special consideration should be given to the elderly or those with physical difficulties to provide parking as near as possible to the clinic they are attending.

Similarly, although doctors may not have the space to provide adequate parking for all patients, special consideration should be given to the elderly and patients with special needs to provide ease of access to health care.

Patients using public transport

Receptionists should be able to inform patients of local bus and train services, and to direct patients to the appropriate pick-up/drop-off points to enable them to reach their destinations. Information about local taxi services should also be available to patients.

Patients using the ambulance service

Receptionists should be aware of the categories of patients eligible for transport by ambulance to and from hospital (walking with assistance, sitting, or stretcher cases). Eligibility is assessed by general practitioners or social services; receptionists will usually be asked by the GP to arrange appropriate transport for the patient's first visit to hospital. Subsequent transport for hospital attendance will either be arranged by the hospital receptionist or secretary, but may also be arranged directly by the hospital's ambulance service administrator.

Total quality in medical practice

The phrase 'total quality' is frequently used without any definition of what total quality actually means for the organization concerned.

NHS trusts, FHSAs and GPs are concerned with providing a quality service to their patients (customers) and many are committed to a total quality programme. An appropriate definition of total quality in providing health care might be:

A cost-effective system for integrating the continuous quality improvement efforts of all involved in health care to deliver services which ensure patient (customer) satisfaction.

Total quality strives to create a climate for excellence

Total quality strives to prevent errors rather than correct them

Total quality is based on effective and harmonious teamwork with absolute commitment of all members of the team

What is a doctor's view of quality?

What is the patient's view?

What is your view?

Patients want easy access to a doctor either in hospital or general practice. They would like to wait in pleasant surroundings and want as short a waiting time as possible. They want a reasonable amount of time set aside for their consultation and expect receptionists and secretaries to smile, be sympathetic and responsive to their needs.

A doctor's perception of quality is probably very different, but they, too, expect an efficient service from their clerical staff as well as from the medical team in providing patient care.

Receptionists, secretaries, nurses and other members of the health team all have a different perception of quality. They cannot be expected to just provide an 'excellent' service while auditing themselves. They must be given the opportunity to share in the vision of what the organization is attempting to achieve. To do the job well, everyone will need guidelines; clear goals and objectives must be set and regular reviews and training given to help them create the climate for excellence.

Team members will be encouraged to set their own objectives and to monitor and improve their individual performance. They should be able to make suggestions for improved working methods and to discuss new ideas for improving the service.

Total quality is an extension of customer care, in which every receptionist and secretary working in the field of health care plays a vital role.

Audit

Audit in health care may be defined as the monitoring and appraisal of performance against predetermined standards and targets to provide a quality service and care for the patient.

Receptionists and secretaries in their day-to-day activities can consider what they do and if they can do it better to provide a quality service to patients.

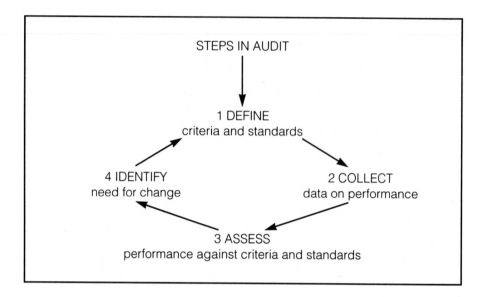

1   Identifying or defining criteria and standards in order to answer the question 'What are we doing/trying to achieve for our patients?'
2   Collecting data on current performance, i.e. the care and/or service given and its effects on patients? Are they satisfied?
3   Assessing performance against criteria to determine whether standards have been met and objectives achieved.
4   Identifying the need for change or improvement in patient care.

The importance of audit

Decision making can only be truly effective when it is based on accurate record keeping and information about various activities, for example, receptionists may be asked to keep records of numbers of patients seen at the surgery or in the hospital clinic. This is important in decision making to improve the quality of care or service to patients:

- to introduce a new clinic

- to extend the length of the surgery or clinic

- to check that the current consultation system is working satisfactorily in the best interests of both doctors and patients

- to increase staffing levels.

Secretaries and receptionists may feel that the information or statistics kept to help decision making is never ending, but it must be remembered that the conclusions drawn may affect all members of the team, and foster a feeling of team spirit and involvement. This in turn will create a professional and caring team playing an important part in the delivery of a high standard of service and health care.

Summary

In this chapter we have looked at the contribution made by both receptionists and secretaries in the health service in their dealings with patients and their role in creating the first impression that patients have of the health care provided both in primary and secondary care.

Quality of health care provision and customer care go hand in hand to achieve ever improving standards and patient satisfaction.

3

Communication

Introduction

Communication is the technical term for passing information. Effective communication is when appropriate information is not only passed on, but seen to be understood and acted upon. Therefore the skills of communication involve:

- listening and understanding what the patient/doctor requires

- conveying appropriate information

- checking that the information has been understood

- checking that a suitable response has been or will be made.

For the medical receptionist the responsibility of communicating with patients is:

to *listen* first

then give *appropriate* information

check by questioning that the patient understands

and *confirm* by observing whether action will be/has been taken whilst *maintaining confidentiality*

Listening

Listening does not merely involve hearing the words that are said, but also hearing what is not said, using intuition, common sense and reading behaviour to get the complete picture. On the telephone this is more difficult because body language (see Chapter 2) cannot be seen. However, it is important to tune into variations in tone of voice. With patients who are well known this will almost be an automatic process, but with people who are new it is even more important to exercise perception to get off to a good start.

The receptionist is the key person in ensuring that information is passed between patients, health care staff, hospitals, general practices, drug company representatives, pharmacists, suppliers, and FHSA/health boards – to name but a few! It is vital that all the communication skills are used to best effect.

The receptionist needs to be skilled in all forms of communication – verbal, written form on paper, or by electronic means – but the majority of a receptionist's time will be spent in verbal communication.

DO	DON'T
Speak clearly	Eat or drink whilst speaking
One thing at a time – give 100% attention to each patient	Do two things at once, e.g. hunt for missing files, or work on the VDU whilst speaking to someone
Use words carefully	Use 'slang' or medical terms to patients
Control conversations with patients – use open and closed questions	Allow the patient to keep you longer than necessary
Be aware of your own tone of voice	Allow anger or frustration to show in your tone of voice

Use of questions in communicating

Awareness of the use of questions can help the receptionist to draw out patient needs or wrap up an unduly lingering conversation. Although a certain amount of questioning will be done automatically, or according to the practice/hospital policy, when difficulty is encountered using the right questions will help.

The simplest classification of questions is that they can be open, closed or leading.

- *Open* questions ease a patient into giving the information that is required, e.g. 'How can I help you ?' encourages the patient to state the need (for an appointment, result of test, etc.).

- *Leading* questions encourage a patient to make a decision by stating alternatives from which one needs to be selected, e.g. 'Do you want the appointment on Monday or Tuesday?' to which the logical answer is one of the two on offer, or 'You want to give up smoking, don't you?' to which the expected answer is 'Yes'.

- *Closed* questions bring the conversation to a halt, e.g. 'Shall I tell the doctor you need to speak to him?' to which the logical answer can only be 'Yes' or 'No'.

OPEN QUESTIONS begin with the words	CLOSED QUESTIONS begin with the words
When . . . . ?	Would you . . . .?
How . . . .?	Shall I . . . .?
Who . . . .?	Are you . . . .?
What . . . .?	Do you . . . .?
Where . . . .?	May I . . . .?

Note: This is why 'May I help you?' is a poor way to address someone when you really want to help them, because the instant answer is either 'No', which is difficult for a British person to say outright to someone they do not know, or 'Yes' but does not help the person formulate their requirement!

Methods of communication

Communication is the way in which we transmit information, knowledge, thoughts and ideas from one person to another or to a group of people. In any organization, large or small, communication is important for the business to function effectively.

The four main methods of communication are:

- the spoken word (direct – face-to-face)

- the written word, e.g. diagrams, posters, notice boards etc.

- the use of telephone systems, including facsimile, answering machines, VDUs, E-mail, etc.

- Non-verbal communication (body language). (See Chapter 2.)

Communication – internal and external

Communication may be either internal or external. The following are examples of written communication.

Written messages

Secretaries and receptionists are always conveying urgent and non-urgent messages from patients or other professionals. It is vital that the messages do not get mislaid and that appropriate action is taken. They should contain:

- the date and time the message is received

- the name, address and telephone number of the caller

- the name of the intended recipient of the message

- a clearly written and concise message

- the name, or initials, of the person taking the message.

Memorandum

A memorandum (memo) is an internal written communication which may be used to convey short messages and information to individuals or to all the health care team. Your organization will, no doubt, use a memorandum form which has several headings.

Notice boards

Notice boards can be used to convey information both internally to the organization or externally to visitors. Notice boards should be positioned so that they are readily visible and accessible to all who are expected to see the notices displayed. Notice boards should be kept up to date, and a member of the team will no doubt have responsibility for this.

White boards

These are often used in organizations to display information relevant to the day. Hospitals and surgeries may display notices about clinics running late, or health promotion information, etc.

Leaflets and posters

Hospitals and surgeries alike have access to a vast quantity of health promotion material and health messages to patients. Managers will often give responsibility to receptionists for displaying leaflets and posters, which should be shown to give impact to the intended message.

Protocols and procedures

All health care organizations will provide written protocols to communicate to members of the team the procedures for the activities in which staff are involved. Written protocols contain standards of quality and should be written so that all members of the team involved in the task fully understand the procedures and thus achieve objectives.

External written communication

Letters remain the most widely used method of written communication. Secretaries will be trained to provide a high standard of letter writing.

Letters are used to communicate with health authorities, NHS trusts, FHSAs, health boards, medical professionals and patients. For example, GPs write referral letters to hospital consultants; hospitals send discharge letters and reports to GPs.

Computers now provide a networking facility linking hospitals, FHSAs, health authorities, laboratories and medical practices.

Telephone skills

Telephone callers only have tone of voice and words to go upon. Any frustrations felt at the time of answering the phone will be conveyed to the caller in the tone of voice and intonation on the words.

It is difficult to illustrate this point from the written word, however, consider the common phrase used by many organizations to answer the telephone: 'How can I help you?' This can be said with a genuine interest, conveyed by a warmth of tone. Alternatively, it can be said in a robotic tone which makes you, the caller, feel as though you want to leave a message on an answer machine for someone else to call back later!

Understandably, by 10.30 am on a busy Monday morning it may be difficult for a stressed receptionist to make an incoming caller feel 'welcome'. Difficult, but not impossible. It may be helpful to have some kind of personal motto to say to oneself at difficult times, e.g. 'Do as you would be done by', 'Speak as you would want to be spoken to'. Self control, conscious use of a warm tone of voice, and the personal motto are useful aids to ensuring the phone is answered to a consistently high standard.

Telephone enquiries

Secretaries and receptionists receive numerous telephone enquiries during the course of their day-to-day work. They may be typing lengthy reports, running a busy surgery or clinic or retrieving data from the computer, but the telephone enquiries and requests continue! Maintaining the balance between conflicting demands is part of the job, and the telephone caller should never have the impression that you are too flustered or annoyed at being interrupted and too busy to deal with their request.

- Answer the telephone as promptly as possible.

- Announce the practice or clinic, and give your name. (You will, no doubt, have your protocol for this.)

- Establish the caller's identity and try to help.

- If the caller is using a pay-phone, take the number and ring them back promptly if necessary.

- Politely ask the caller to hold if you need to deal with a visitor.

Golden rules when using the telephone

- Be polite.

- Do not eat while you are speaking on the telephone.

- Do not hold two conversations at the same time.

- Return to the caller every 30 seconds if you are keeping them on hold.

- If you are unable to help the caller yourself, track down someone who can – if necessary call them back.

People skills – face-to-face

In contrast to telephone communication where the only indicators are words and tone of voice, in a face-to-face encounter there is the additional dimension of 'non-verbal communication'. These are the signals that are given out and picked up, sometimes subconsciously, but which cause a reaction every bit as strong as to the words and tone. For example, a patient who is failing to get what they want is not only likely to raise their voice, but lean forwards over the reception counter. In response a receptionist could either spontaneously lean forward with a matching aggressive reaction, step back from the desk in a defensive manner, or calmly remain in the same position. Not only does the body move and thereby speak more clearly than our words, but the hands and face under-line the expression of feeling. Hands may become clenched into fists and miles disappear. With this knowledge in mind, the skill is to maintain self control and gain control of the situation. There are no set patterns of dealing with difficult situations, but attending courses, practice in role play, watching video clips, discussing situations after they have happened, watching colleagues and learning from their successes/weak-nesses can all contribute to gaining experience and improving existing skills.

The medical receptionist or secretary also needs to constantly bear in mind the fact that patients are likely to not feel well, be anxious about what is going to be done to them, what the doctor may say, and concerned about the effect of their illness on the family. These feelings make patients stressed and therefore more sensitive to off-hand treatment. From the moment they are dealt with they need to feel that they are the one and only concern of the receptionist.

Recall good and bad experiences of how you have been made to feel in shops, offices, hospital, doctor's surgery

What made you feel bad?

What made you feel good?

What can you incorporate into your way of working to make patients feel as good as they can in the circumstances?

Meetings

Staff meetings, departmental or primary health care team meetings and patient participation groups are the type of meeting where receptionists and secretaries may be required to express a view. With modern management techniques meetings have become an important tool for communicating. They are the opportunity to find out what is going on, to be updated with the latest information, and to contribute to forward planning. Even in a well-chaired, relatively informal meeting, staff who have every confidence in dealing with difficult patients at the desk may find it almost impossible to speak out in a meeting with doctors/managers present. The skill to speak out can be cultivated by practice, and helped by planning.

If you are going to be called upon to speak, prepare for the occasion

DO

Read the agenda circulated a few days before the meeting

Think about what you want to say

Write down a few key words

Define one statement that encapsulates your view succinctly

Make an outline of what you want to say

You should succeed in confidently making your point and gain respect not only for your view but for your ability to communicate

DON'T

Go into the meeting intending to say whatever comes into your head at the time

You may lose the opportunity to say what you really want to say, waste other people's time, and they may lose respect for you

---

Performance review

Receptionists and secretaries will no doubt be aware of other forms of 'communication' within their organizations, for example, performance review or 'appraisal' interviews, where he/she will be given the opportunity to communicate how they perceive their personal strengths and limitations, and perhaps identify areas where further training is needed.

Counselling

Counselling may be defined as: 'assisting individuals towards indepen-dence or self-actualization'. It is a form of communication designed to enable employees to make their own decisions or choices. It involves:

- listening

- guiding

- communicating

- information giving.

Counselling is non-judgemental, it does not make assumptions, and can be used to prevent a problem, or can help to work through an existing problem.

The practice leaflet

Practice information leaflets communicate to patients the services avail-able at the practice and how they may make better use of the primary health care service. New patients will find the practice leaflet a valuable source of information, not only about the services offered, but also regard-ing the members of the primary health care team, the times of the surgery and clinic sessions and how to contact the doctor in an emergency.

Your practice leaflets should be attractively designed to make both patients and potential patients aware of the services and quality of care provided. They should be prominently positioned on the reception counter and readily accessible to all callers.

Hospital information leaflets

NHS trusts and private hospitals and clinics will provide information about the services which they offer. As well as basic information of hospi-tal clinics, open access facilities, and times of visiting, etc., they will give details of transport to the hospital and car-parking provision.

Networking

Every organization is changing to a greater or lesser degree on a regular basis. Staff come and go, the organizational structure changes, responsibilities are shifted from one department to another. Therefore it is important that personal contacts are made and maintained so that if a receptionist/secretary does not know how to do something, or does not have a vital piece of information, then there is always someone to turn to, who will either know the answer themselves, or 'know a man who does'. It is also important to keep up to date with the latest information by reading magazines as a vital supplement to networking.

Barriers to communication

Physical barriers

Physical barriers to communication may include the following:

- too much noise
- insufficient privacy
- frequent interruptions
- physical handicap, e.g. deafness, blindness, or stammer
- the reception counter may be too high or too low
- telephone constantly ringing.

Receptionists'/secretaries' language

The language used when speaking to patients is a vital part of good communication. You must be aware of:

- using words (and 'jargon') that the patient cannot understand
- talking too quickly, or too quietly
- talking with a strong accent
- confusing patients by giving them too much information.

Patients' language

Patients from ethnic minorities may have difficulty in understanding and speaking the English language. You may have a colleague who can speak their language, or an interpreter may be necessary.

Psychological barriers

You must be aware of the psychological elements which may form barriers to good communication. Patients may find it difficult to communicate for the following reasons:

- feelings of inadequacy
- lacking in confidence
- emotionally upset by pain and/or anxiety about their medical condition
- unable to concentrate because of illness.

Attitudes of secretaries and receptionists

Remember the importance of positive non-verbal signs. A negative attitude will be a barrier to communication, for example:

- impatience and rudeness
- may not give undivided attention
- appear critical or demonstrate a superior attitude
- lack of eye contact
- appear to be too busy
- feeling cross and under stress.

Attitudes of patients

An understanding of the reasons for patients' attitudes may help you to deal with them in a sympathetic manner and to overcome the barrier their attitude may present. For example they may be:

- too ill to concentrate

- resentful at having to present themselves at the reception desk

- terrified they have a serious illness

- afraid of appearing stupid to the efficient secretary or receptionist

- have a personal problem

- inhibited by finding they know the receptionist or secretary socially.

Overcoming the barriers

An awareness of the barriers combined with good common sense is a good start to overcoming any problems.

- Try to answer all questions in a positive way.

- A pleasant manner, a smile and understanding often does the trick – it is hard to be difficult when empathy is extended to you.

- Always be polite.

- Be alert to any problems which might occur.

- Always try to be helpful, smiling, calm and able to cope.

- If patients are kept waiting for longer than necessary, apologize, and give an explanation.

- When making appointments, ensure that the patients have the date and time written down to avoid any future misunderstanding.

- Try to give each patient your attention when dealing with them. Make eye contact, listen carefully to what they are saying.

- Never sound tired, or bored or look as if you are not listening.

Confidentiality

Remember that the rules of confidentiality that apply to working in any health care environment are as equally important when communicating with patients.

All information is privileged information, and *must not* be divulged without the doctor's prior consent.

4

Law, ethics and medicine

Introduction

The relationships between professional health care workers and between them and their patients are governed by the professional ethics and etiquette of medicine which have developed over the centuries together with developments in medicine itself. Secretaries and receptionists working closely with doctors and other health care workers, as well as being in constant communication with patients, should be aware of the important role of ethics and etiquette.

Ethics relate to moral principles and standards of what is morally right and wrong and are the guiding rules of professional behaviour. They are directed towards the benefit of the patients. *Etiquette* is concerned with the courtesy and politeness of normal behaviour.

History of ethics and etiquette

History shows that even from the earliest times, various legal systems have incorporated some degree of regulation of doctors. The earliest records were the Code of Laws of Hammurabi (1790 BC), when fees were regulated. Success was rewarded in accordance with the status of the patient, but failure was punished, frequently by mutilation.

The earliest record and declaration of ethics was made in the Hippocratic Oath (400 BC), which reflects the culture of the Hippocratic physicians. The standards expressed in the Hippocratic Oath, although no longer affirmed by today's physicians, is still accepted as the ideal of professional behaviour. (See Appendix 2.)

The Hippocratic Oath demonstrates the early concern of the profession to regulate itself by laying down basic standards of professional conduct, not only between doctor and patient, but also between teacher and pupil. For centuries thereafter, the principles of Christian humanism dominated the practice of medicine. Traditions of etiquette in public and private life gradually came about, and, combined with the criteria of professional conduct, established the physician's position in society.

In 1798, the proposals of Sir Thomas Percival in Manchester ultimately became the 'Professional Conduct of Physicians and Surgeons', published in 1803. This laid the foundations for modern ethical standards in the UK.

The Provincial Medical and Surgical Association formed in 1832, which became the British Medical Association (BMA) in 1856, appointed a committee on medical ethics in 1849. This formed the basis of the General Ethical Committee of the BMA which has always played a leading role not only establishing ethical standards for the professional in the UK, but also for standards adopted as norms of conduct for doctors in many parts of the world.

The BMA was largely responsible for the establishment of the General Medical Council (GMC) under the Medical Act of 1858. The GMC has a regulatory role and from time to time issues guidance to members of the medical profession to enable them to avoid action which might lead to charges of professional misconduct. (The roles of both the BMA and GMC will be covered in more detail later in this chapter.)

Medical ethics and etiquette

Every medical receptionist and secretary must be aware of the important areas of ethical behaviour and etiquette. It has already been stated that ethics are directed towards the benefits of the patients, and many are bound into a code of conduct published by the GMC for doctors, and by other regulatory bodies for other health professionals, for example:

- General Dental Council – Dentists
- General Nursing Council – Nurses.

All regulatory bodies have the responsibility of maintaining the register of those allowed to practise as a doctor, dentist, nurse, etc. The ultimate sanction of those judged to have behaved unethically is the removal of their name from the register, and thus the removal of the ability to practise.

There are no formal sanctions for those in breach of etiquette, but the rules have been established by custom. They aid communication between professionals and avoid damaging reputations, so they may be said to indirectly benefit patients.

A modern restatement of the Hippocratic Oath was formulated by the World Medical Association in 1947 to reflect the changing attitudes of society and major advances in medical science. It is known as the Declaration of Geneva:

> I solemnly pledge myself to consecrate my life to the service of humanity;
> I will give to my teachers the respect and gratitude which is their due;
> I will practise my profession with dignity;
> The health of my patient will be my first consideration;
> I will respect the secrets which are confided in me, even after the patient has died;
> I will maintain by all the means of my power, the honour and the noble traditions of the medical profession;
> My colleagues will be my brothers;
> I will not permit considerations of religion, nationality, race, party politics or social standing to intervene between me and my patients;
> I will maintain the utmost respect for human life from the time of conception; even under threat I will not use my medical knowledge contrary to the laws of humanity;
> I make these promises solemnly, freely and upon my honour.

There are four important areas of ethical behaviour and etiquette that all secretaries and receptionists in medical practice should be aware of and should apply the principles of to their day-to-day work:

- confidentiality
- trust
- confidence
- integrity.

Confidentiality

Confidentiality places a constraint upon all those who work in the field of health care. The terms and conditions of employment of medical secretaries and receptionists, wherever employed, will almost certainly contain a clause to the effect that any breach of confidentiality will result in disciplinary action, even dismissal; they will, no doubt, be asked to sign statements signifying that this is fully understood.

The Declaration of Geneva maintains that a doctor must preserve secrecy in all he knows – even after the death of his patient. However, there are certain exceptions to this:

- when the patient gives consent

- when it is undesirable on medical grounds to seek a patient's consent, but it is in the patient's best interests that confidentiality should be broken

- the doctor's overriding duty to society

- for the purposes of medical research, when approved by a local clinical research ethical committee, or in the case of the National Cancer Registry by the Chairman of the BMA's Central Ethical Committee.

Doctors must be able to justify their decisions to disclose information. A doctor must ensure, as far as possible, that all medical information is kept in a secure place.

Confidentiality and medical records

Secretaries and receptionists are in the privileged position of having access to medical records which contain confidential information about patients and they should always remember that patients trust doctors not to divulge any personal information contained in the record. Likewise, confidential information should never be discussed or divulged by secretaries or receptionists.

Discretion is necessary when dealing with enquiries from solicitors, relatives or representatives of the patient, and insurance companies. Staff should always be circumspect when they deal with patients. When speaking with colleagues, great care should be taken. Some hospitals insist that patients are referred to by their hospital number and not by name.

Secretaries and receptionists working in a hospital will usually find that their medical records manager will require them to sign a form stating that they understand the legal and ethical aspects of confidentiality and that any behaviour contravening this may result in termination of employment.

Any information contained in medical records may only be disclosed in certain circumstances.

Trust

Doctors as part of their work in dealing with patients and their families are entrusted with information that would not be divulged to others. Good medical practice is based on the maintenance of trust between doctors, patients and their families with the knowledge that professional relationships will be strictly observed. Not only doctors, but medical secretaries and receptionists must at all times exercise care and discretion to maintain this special relationship.

Confidence

Confidence like trust is also vitally important in the doctor/patient relationship. Staff should appreciate that if patients have been helped by a doctor on a previous occasion, they are confident they will be helped in any further episodes. Whilst this may make the doctor's task easier, it also places added responsibility on the doctor – doctors know they can not always succeed.

Integrity

Doctors will act professionally and objectively in the best interests of their patients in their judgements and patient care. Receptionists and staff also should behave in a professional manner and remain circumspect at all times. Considerable pressure is placed on doctors and health care staff, for example pressures from relatives, advertising, the media, etc. It is, perhaps, worth considering the duties of a doctor and rights of patients in the context of ethics and etiquette in medicine.

Doctors' duties

Duties of a doctor in general

- A doctor must always maintain the highest standards of medical conduct.
- A doctor must practise their profession uninfluenced by motives of profit.

Duties of a doctor to the sick

- A doctor must always bear in mind the obligation of preserving human life.
- A doctor owes the patient complete loyalty and all the resources of their service.
- A doctor shall preserve absolute secrecy on all they know about their patients because of the confidence entrusted in them.

- A doctor must give emergency care as a humanitarian duty unless they are assured that others are willing and able to give such care.

- Whenever an examination or treatment is beyond their capacity they should summon another doctor who has the necessary ability.

- A doctor must act without discrimination or motive of profit regardless of race, colour or creed.

Overall management

It is good medical practice for one doctor to be responsible for the overall management of a patient's illness.

Referral from a GP to a consultant has evolved in the patient's interest. A consultant or specialist should not accept a patient without referral from a GP. There are exceptions, e.g. sexually transmitted diseases, family planning, and casualty.

Consent to treatment

The patient's trust that their consent to treatment will not be misused is an essential part of their relationship with their doctor; for a doctor even to touch a patient without consent is an assault. Doctors offer advice, but it is the patient who decides whether or not to accept the advice. The onus is on the doctor to explain in such a way that advice will be accepted.

Patients' rights

Patients have certain rights in relation to their use of health care services. These rights generally fall into two categories:

1   the right to treatment
2   the right to confidentiality.

The right to treatment

A patient:

- has the right to be on a GP's list of patients

- has the right to see a GP (not necessarily their own) at the GP's surgery at any time during surgery hours

- should have access to a telephone number at which a GP can be reached 24 hours a day, 365 days a year

- should be visited at home if it is considered necessary by the GP

- must receive any treatment which is immediately necessary when temporarily away from home

- has the right to change GPs without giving a reason by applying to another GP

- has no absolute right to a second opinion, but the doctor should take reasonable care to seek one if they are unsure of the diagnosis or treatment

- needs to give consent before being examined or treated

- is not legally bound to accept treatment. However, doctors can give essential treatment if the patient is temporarily incapable of understanding or consenting to treatment, e.g. through alcohol or drugs. If the patient is permanently incapable through mental illness it is possible for a legal guardian to give consent

- has the right to refuse to be examined with a medical student present

- has the right to a full and truthful reply to any specific question unless the information may result in anxiety which may injure the patient's health

- has the right to see and amend medical records made on or after 1 November 1991, unless they will cause harm to the patient. (See Access to Health Records Act 1990.) Hospitals, private clinics, GP practices, etc. who hold patient information on computer have to follow the Data Protection Act which protects patients' rights (Data Protection Act 1984)

- has the right to complain about their doctor if they have not followed their terms of service or if a doctor behaves in an unethical manner.

The right to confidentiality

Doctors must not pass on information without the patient's consent except to those involved in the treatment and care, or, when it is in the best interests of the patient, to close relatives. The law requires doctors to give information about patients to health and other authorities in certain circumstances:

- when ordered by a court
- if the patient has certain infectious diseases or food poisoning
- if they suspect the patient is addicted to a hard drug
- if they arrange an abortion for a patient
- if required by the police to help identify a driver suspected of motoring offences.

Chaperoning

All too frequently we hear about doctors accused of indecently assaulting their patients, and doctors today are at risk from such accusations. The presence of a third person as a chaperone, usually a nurse, is a valuable insurance for the practitioner. However, there may be occasions when the doctor's secretary or receptionist will be asked to be present at the consultation, particularly in private practice when a nurse is not always available.

If the patient is emotionally upset or mentally disturbed when consulting a doctor, the presence of a chaperone not only protects the doctor, but may also relieve the patient of some embarrassment and anxiety.

The regulatory bodies and their role

The General Medical Council

The General Medical Council (GMC) was established under the Medical Act of 1858 with the purpose of distinguishing between unqualified practitioners or 'quacks' and the qualified medical practitioner. The Medical Register was thus established, with records of medical practitioners and their qualifications.

Functions of the GMC

- To keep a register of all medical practitioners who have obtained qualifying degrees, giving them licence to practise.

- To keep a separate register of those practitioners who have obtained higher degrees.

- The GMC sets out standards of medical education.

- It is responsible for the publication of the British Pharmacopoeia (BP).

- The GMC has an important regulatory role; it issues guidelines to all members of the medical profession to enable them to avoid actions which might lead to charges of professional misconduct.

- It has a duty to administer discipline. It is to the GMC that the public and medical profession may make complaints about a doctor's behaviour.

- The GMC has the power, if such a charge is proved, to temporarily suspend a doctor from practising, or, if necessary, to remove their name ('struck-off') from the register.

The British Medical Association

The British Medical Association (BMA) was founded in 1832 by Charles Hastings and is the largest medical association in the UK. It is concerned with most aspects of medicine and is one of the principal bodies representing British doctors.

The BMA played an important part in the establishment of the General Medical Council. The Central Ethical Committee of the BMA plays a leading role in establishing ethical standards for the medical profession in the UK, and also for the standards which have been adopted as norms of conduct for doctors throughout the world.

Medical science is advancing so rapidly and with new discoveries being communicated to the public, the BMA issues ethical guidelines to reflect and safeguard the well-being and interests of patients, and, at the same time, expressing the views of the profession on medical ethics.

Summary of medical ethics and etiquette

In looking at the ethics and etiquette of medical practice, the receptionist or secretary will understand that patients not only expect doctors to use their expertise and skill, but also to observe absolute confidentiality regarding any information imparted as a result of the consultation, examination and treatment. On this understanding of professional confidence and secrecy, all those working in the field of health care will be aware of the special relationship which exists between doctor and patient.

Having considered the various ethical issues that confront the medical profession, and the role of the regulatory bodies, we are able to appreciate the problems facing doctors and their ability to resolve the numerous ethical and moral dilemmas that may arise. These include:

- abortion

- euthanasia

- screening

- genetic counselling

- artificial insemination

- severely malformed infants

- in vitro fertilization

- consent to operations on reproductive organs

- HIV/AIDS.

Practical considerations for secretaries and receptionists

- Remember that your work is strictly confidential – anything that is divulged by a patient to the doctor, the medical records or correspondence must not be disclosed to anyone else.

- Details of your work or personal affairs of doctors and other health care professionals must *not* be discussed.

- The behaviour of, or treatment by, a medical practitioner or any professional health care worker must *not* be openly criticized within hearing distance of the patient.

- Always be circumspect when talking about a doctor or other health care professional to another person. Do not unduly praise or criticize their accomplishments.

- It is your responsibility to facilitate the doctor's treatment and care of their patients.

Legal aspects

Medical secretaries and receptionists, although not needing detailed knowledge of law, should have an understanding of those legal aspects affecting their day-to-day work.

Medical Records

Hospitals, general practice and any health care organization recording information on computer about identifiable living individuals must ensure that the provisions of the Data Protection Act are complied with.

The Data Protection Act 1984

The Data Protection Act is designed and based on principles to ensure that information relating to an individual is obtained fairly, kept up to date and stored securely. Individuals, whose data are stored, have rights of access enabling them to check the accuracy of the information. The data protection registrar and the courts are empowered to require correction of inaccurate material if it is not undertaken voluntarily by the data user.

The medical context of the individual's right of access to information held about him/her has been modified by the Data Protection (Subject Access Modification) (Health) Order 1987. This allows information to be withheld from an individual if it is likely to cause serious harm to his or her mental or physical health, or discloses the identity of another person other than the health care professional. A doctor who withholds information must be prepared to justify their actions in a court if challenged at a later date. This Act applies to England, Wales, Scotland and Northern Ireland.

The Access to Medical Reports Act 1988

This Act establishes an individual's right of access to medical reports prepared for insurance or employment purposes, by doctors who, either are, or have been, responsible for that person's care. The Act applies only to England, Wales and Scotland, but similar provisions now apply to Northern Ireland under the Access to Personal Files and Medical Reports Order 1991.

At the same time that the patient's consent to the preparation of the report is obtained, the commissioning company is required to inform the individual of his/her rights under the Act, and to enquire whether access to the report is required. The information is passed on to the doctor.

If the patient requires access, he/she is allowed 21 days to make appropriate arrangements to view the report. Patients who originally declined the opportunity of access may make application to see the report until the time it is despatched to the company, and if so, must be allowed 21 days to make appropriate arrangements.

Once the report has been seen by the patient, he/she may agree to the despatch unaltered, request correction of factual accuracy, or where the doctor declines to make the requested correction, append a statement of his/her own, or may refuse to allow the report to be released.

The Access to Health Records Act 1990

This Act applies to England, Wales and Scotland and has established a right of access for patients to whom the records relate and, in certain circumstances, to other individuals. The Act also makes provision for correction of inaccurate records.

Under the Act, a health record is any record containing information relating to the physical or mental health of an individual who can be identified from that information which has been made by 'or on behalf of' a health care professional.

Applications for access must be made in writing to the record holder and, provided no addition to the record has been made within the previous 40 days, a fee may be charged. Provided there is no reason to withhold access, the record holder must allow the applicant to see the records within 40 days, unless the most recent note has been made within 40 days, in which case the time limit is 21 days. If a copied set of the medical record is required, a copying and postal charge may be made. Applications may be made by the patient or someone appointed on the patient's behalf:

- in the case of a child, the parent or guardian

- in the case of an incapable patient, a person appointed by the court to manage their affairs

- after a patient's death, by the patient's personal representatives or anyone who might have a claim arising out of the patient's death.

The Law and Mental Health

Mental Health Act

Secretaries and receptionists working in the field of health care will need an understanding of the implications of the law relating to mental illness.

The law has changed with the Mental Health Act of 1983. The provisions of this Act are of particular importance to those patients who are compulsorily detained under the Act. This involves approximately 10% of all patients who are admitted to psychiatric hospitals or departments.

The Mental Health Act of 1983 established the Mental Health Act Commission which has a responsibility to protect the rights of detained patients and to keep under review the exercise of compulsory power and duties conferred by the Act. The Act also provides the legal instrument which enables society to act in the interests of, and on behalf of, patients and those convicted of certain criminal offences, who are diagnosed as having certain abnormal mental conditions, and makes provision for the protection of the public, and for the protection of the property of patients compulsorily detained.

The primary concerns of the 1983 Mental Health Act are:

- protection of the mentally sick person
- protection of his/her property
- protection of the public.

The Act defines certain relevant legal mental conditions as follow.

- *Mental disorder* which means illness, arrested or incomplete development of mind, psychopathic disorder and any other disorder or disability of mind.

- *Severe mental impairment* which means a state of arrested or incomplete development of intelligence and social functions, and is associated with abnormally aggressive or seriously irresponsible conduct on the part of the person concerned.

- *Mental impairment* which means a state of arrested or incomplete development of mind (not amounting to severe mental impairment) which includes significant impairment of intelligence and social functioning and is associated with abnormally aggressive or seriously irresponsible conduct on the part of the person concerned.

- *Psychopathic disorder* which means a persistent disorder or disability of mind (whether or not including significant impairment of intelligence) which results in abnormally aggressive or seriously irresponsible conduct on the part of the person concerned.

A person may not be regarded as suffering from mental disorder by reason only of promiscuity or other immoral conduct, sexual deviancy or dependence on alcohol or drugs.

The legislation emphazises:

1   As much treatment as possible on a voluntary basis, both in hospital and in the home or other institution.
2   A shift from institutional care to care within the home as far as possible.
3   Proper provision for those to be detained on a compulsory basis in the interests of the patient and society.

Medical secretaries and receptionists will from time to time be involved in arrangements for patient admission, either formally or informally, to undergo psychiatric treatment. Such admissions come within sections of the Mental Health Act. A brief outline of admission under some of the sections of the Mental Health Act is given on the following page.

Methods by which a person may enter a hospital for psychiatric treatment

Informal admission (Section 131)

Any person having attained the age of 16 may request admission, or a person under the age of 16 where the parent or guardian gives consent, or any person to whom it is suggested that admission is advisable and that person does not refuse, can be admitted without any legal formalities. This patient can discharge him/herself unless the doctor in charge decides that if discharged he/she would be endangering his/her health or safety or that of others.

Compulsory admission and detention

The following methods of admission can be used when a person suffering from mental disorder as defined by the Act is in need of psychiatric care but is not prepared to enter hospital or remain in hospital for observation or treatment.

- *Section 2: (up to 28 days)* – Admission for assessment (or for assessment followed by medical treatment).
  An application for the admission of the patient must be made either by an approved social worker or the nearest relative, plus a medical recommendation from one 'psychiatrist' and a doctor (if practicable one doctor should have previous acquaintance of the patient, for example, his/her GP). The person making the application should have seen the patient within the last 14 days.

- *Section 3: (up to 6 months)* – Detention for treatment.
  The application for detention under Section 3 is the same as for Section 2, except that the approved social worker is not to act if the nearest relative objects. This section can be reviewed for a further six months, and yearly thereafter.

  Note: Patients may apply to the Mental Health Review Tribunal (NHRT) under Sections 2 and 3, subject to the stated criteria.

- *Section 4: (up to 72 hours)* – Admission for assessment.
  The application must be made either by an approved social worker or the nearest relative, plus a recommendation from a medical practitioner who must have seen the patient within the last 24 hours. The patient must arrive at the hospital within 24 hours of the medical examination. (This may be converted into Section 2 if a second medical recommendation is received within 72 hours.)

Consent to treatment

Certain sections (56 – 64) of the Mental Health Act are largely concerned with consent to treatment for long-term detained patients, but certain safeguards also apply to informal patients.

Employment law

There are a number of laws influencing the employment of staff, of which the Employment Protection (Consolidation) Act of 1978 is probably the most relevant. It is important that all employees, including medical secretaries and receptionists, understand their rights.

From the point when a verbal offer of a job has been made and the post accepted, the formal contract comes into being. At this stage nothing further is required to signify its existence and both parties are bound by it from that point on. However, to avoid any misunderstanding, employers will generally follow up a job offer and acceptance with a letter.

Written statement of main terms and conditions

New legislation came into effect in November 1993, requiring employers to give new employees working eight hours or more each week, a written statement of the main terms and conditions of their employment within two months of starting. Prior to November 1993, a written statement was only required for those working 16 hours or more per week, and staff working between eight and 16 hours only became eligible after five years. If existing eligible staff request it, they must be given a written statement within two months of asking. They must be notified of any changes to specified terms and conditions when they occur, even if they have not requested a written statement.

The written statement must contain:

- the employer's name
- the employee's name
- starting date of employment
- date continuous service began and whether or not employment with another employer (other hospital or medical practice) is counted
- job title
- rate of pay
- payment intervals (monthly, weekly)

- hours of work

- place of work

- holiday entitlement and holiday pay.

The following additional information must also be provided within the two-month period (as part of the principal statement or separately):

- sick leave and sick pay

- pension scheme

- notice periods on either side

- end date of a fixed-term contract, or likely end date of a temporary one

- particulars of collective agreements where these apply (e.g. as agreed by Whitley Council)

- grievance procedure and to whom a grievance can be raised

- disciplinary rules and procedures, and to whom appeals can be made – this applies only to employers of 20 or more staff.

Sometimes relevant information relating to sickness, pensions, grievances, disciplinary rules, procedures and appeals is kept in separate reference documents. In this case, the written statement will refer to these; they should be readily accessible to employees in the course of their work.

Equality of opportunity

We discriminate between people both in the workplace and in day-to-day life. Some forms of discrimination are acceptable, but others are not, and certain forms have been determined to be unlawful. Legislation relating to equality of opportunity requires employers to exercise some form of social responsibility in making decisions about employees, current or potential. Employees, too, may unconsciously discriminate between people; we are not always aware of how our prejudices and preconceptions colour our judgement and the way we deal with others.

Equality can only be achieved through an acceptance by all members of the work team that it is important, in their own interests and in the interests of the service they provide.

Equal opportunities legislation

Equality of opportunity regardless of sex, race, marriage, disablement, religion or age is vitally important, not only for employees to have a fair/equal chance of developing their potential abilities and realizing their expectations, but also for employers to make full and effective use of their staff and to improve employee relations. This legislation forbids discrimination between men and women with regard to pay and other terms in their contracts, for example:

- *Equal Pay Act 1970 and Equal Pay (Amendments) Regulations 1983*

    – overtime
    – bonus payments
    – holiday and sick pay entitlements.

- *Rehabilitation of Offenders Act 1974*

This Act allows an individual who has had a conviction for an offence to put it behind them and be rehabilitated after a period of time. Their conviction becomes 'spent' and they may lawfully conceal it from a prospective employer, as if it had never happened. However, certain exemptions exist.

- *Sex Discrimination Act 1975*

The Act describes direct discrimination as occurring if, on the grounds of her sex, a woman is treated less favourably than a man would be treated.

- *The Race Relations Act 1976*

The Act forbids racial discrimination in employment. It states that no person should treat another less favourably on racial grounds.

- *Disabled Persons (Employment) Act 1944*

This Act places a duty upon employers with more than 20 workers to employ a quota (currently 3%) of employees registered as disabled according to the terms of the Act.

General responsibilities under these Acts

Hospitals, medical practices, etc. have a legal obligation to ensure that they and their employees do not discriminate unlawfully.

All supervisory staff are responsible for eliminating any sexual harassment, victimization or intimidation of which they are aware.

Individual employees are expected to co-operate with measures designed to ensure equal opportunities and avoid unlawful discrimination. They should be encouraged to report incidents of harassment, victimization and pressure to discriminate where these occur.

Sexual harassment

Sexual harassment is judged as unlawful behaviour contrary to the Sex Discrimination Act 1974. Examples of sexual harassment are:

- unwanted physical conduct
- requests for sexual favours
- unwelcome sexual advances
- continued suggestions for social activity outside of work after it has been made clear that such suggestions are not welcome
- offensive flirtation, suggestive remarks, etc.
- the display of pornographic or sexually suggestive pictures, etc.
- leering, whistling or making sexually suggestive gestures
- derogatory or degrading abuse or insults which are gender related
- offensive comments about appearance or dress.

Certification

All doctors, whether working in private practices or in an NHS organization are requested from time to time to issue certificates, including:

- National Insurance/DSS certificates
- death certificates
- cremation certificates
- private medical or insurance certificates
- certificates of stillbirth.

Certification is a statutory obligation imposed upon doctors, and the secretary or receptionist should do all they can to ensure that the doctor is not placed in the position of being asked to improperly certify.

For example the doctor must always see the patient when issuing and signing the form on which a patient claims sickness benefit – Form Med 3 (Figures 4.1 and 4.2). This should not be issued more than one day after examination as the doctor has to certify that they have examined the patient today/yesterday.

FOR SOCIAL SECURITY AND STATUTORY SICK PAY PURPOSES ONLY

<u>NOTES TO PATIENT ABOUT USING THIS FORM</u>

You can use this form either:

    1.   For Statutory Sick Pay (SSP) purposes - fill in Part A overleaf. Also fill in Part B if the doctor has given you a date to resume work. Give or send the completed form to your employer.

    2.   For Social Security purposes -
To continue a claim for state benefit fill in Parts A and C of the form overleaf. Also fill in Part B if the doctor has given you a date to resume work. **Sign and date the form and give or send it to your Local Social Security Office QUICKLY to avoid losing benefit.**

NOTE: To start your claim for State benefit you must use form SC1 if you are self-employed, unemployed or non-employed OR form SSP1 if you are an employee. For further details get leaflet NI16 (from Social Security Local Offices).

Doctor's Statement

In confidence to

Mr/Mrs/Miss/Ms ....

I examined you today/yesterday and advised you that

(a) You need not   (b) you should refrain from work
    refrain from
    work   for*†...

                OR until ....

Diagnosis of your disorder
causing absence from work ....
Doctor's remarks

Doctor's   Date of
signature   signing

Form Med 3

NOTE TO DOCTOR*†   *See inside front cover for notes on completion*

Printed in the UK for HMSO 03/94 D.8444690 C50.000. 36625. (T3453)

Figure 4.1   Form Med 3 (sample).

if you cannot fill this in yourself ask someone to do so and sign it for you.

A.   TO BE COMPLETED IN ALL CASES - PLEASE USE BLOCK LETTERS

Surname Mr/Mrs/Miss/Ms

First names

Present address

Postcode

	Date	Month	Year
Date of birth			

National Insurance
Number

Works or Clock Number
or Department

B.   If the doctor has given you a date to resume work

Date you intend to start
(or seek) work for any
employer or as a self-
employed person

day   Date   Month   Year

For night shift
workers only

Shift will begin at   Time   am/pm

and end next day at   Time   am/pm

C.   FOR STATE BENEFIT CLAIMANTS ONLY

Full name and address
of employer (if employed)

DECLARATION

I understand that if I give incorrect or incomplete information action may be taken against me.

I declare that because of incapacity I have not worked since the date of my last claim.

I also declare that my circumstances and those of my dependants are and have been as last stated. (If there has been a change cross out this declaration and attach a signed and dated statement of new facts.)

I declare that the information I have given on this form is correct and complete.

I agree that a doctor acting on behalf of the Department of Social Security may get in touch with my doctor so that they may give the Department of Social Security any information which is needed to deal with this claim and any request to look at the claim again.

Signature .... Date ....

If you have signed this form for someone else
please tick here

Figure 4.1   *Continued*

FOR SOCIAL SECURITY AND STATUTORY   **Special Statement**
SICK PAY PURPOSES ONLY   **by the Doctor**

In confidence to
Mr/Mrs/Miss/Ms..

(A) I examined you on the   (B) I have not examined you but, on the basis of
                                   a recent written report from –

following dates ....   Doctor .... (Name if known)

....   of ....

....
and advised you that you
should refrain from work   .... (Address)
                                   I have advised you that you should refrain

from .... to ....   from work for/until ....

Diagnosis of your disorder
causing absence from work ....
Doctor's remarks

Doctor's   Date of
signature   signing

*The special circumstances in which this form may be used are described in the
handbook "Medical Evidence for Social Security and Statutory Sick Pay Purposes".*

Form Med 5
3/83

PATIENT TO COMPLETE PARTICULARS ON REVERSE

Figure 4.2   Form Med 5.

TO BE COMPLETED IN ALL CASES – PLEASE USE BLOCK LETTERS
If you cannot fill this form in yourself, ask someone else to do so

Surname Mr/Mrs/Miss/Ms

First names

Present address

| | Postcode |

| Date of birth | Date | Month | Year |

National insurance number

Works or clock number
or department

If the doctor has given you a date to resume work
date you intend to start (or
seek) work for an employer
or as a self-employed person

day   Date   Month   Year

| For night shift workers only | Shift will begin at and end next day at | Time   am/pm |
| | | Time   am/pm |

FOR STATE BENEFIT CLAIMANTS ONLY
If you wish to claim benefit, continue below. To avoid losing benefit send this form
QUICKLY to your local Social Security Office.
NOTE: To start your claim for State benefit you must use form SC1 (Rev) if you are
self-employed, unemployed or non-employed OR form SSP1(E) or SSP1(T) if you
are an employee. For further details get leaflet N16 (from DHSS local offices).

Full name and address
of employer (if employed)

DECLARATION

Remember: if you give information that is incorrect or incomplete action may be
taken against you.
I declare that because of incapacity I have not worked since the date of my last
claim. I also declare that my circumstances and those of my dependants are and
have been as last stated. (If there has been a change cross out this declaration and
attach a signed and dated statement of new facts).
I declare that the information I have given is correct and complete.
I claim benefit.
I agree to my doctor giving medical information relevant to my claim to a doctor in
the Regional Medical Service.
**Sign
here** .... Date ....
If you have signed on behalf of the person
claiming tick the box.

Printed in the UK for HMSO 7/87 Dd. 8080423 C 2,550 (11037).

Figure 4.2 *Continued*

Death certificates

The death certificate is the oldest of all official medical forms and is issued only to registered practitioners. The certificate is obtained from the registrar for the subdistrict in which the doctor practises. The issue of death certificates is a statutory requirement and no fee is chargeable. The certificate is given by a doctor who was actually attending the patient in their last illness, and where there is sufficient knowledge of the cause of death to do so. Doctors are bound by law to provide the certificate in a sealed envelope. The death certificate should be taken to the Registrar of Births and Deaths in the subdistrict of occurrence within five days of death.

There is no legal duty to notify the coroner of any death, but of course, this does not imply that the doctor need not do so when the circumstances require such action. Moral, ethical and traditional considerations necessitate that the doctor acts with responsibility and, by notifying the coroner, facilitates any enquiry into the death as the coroner deems advisable.

Role of medical secretary or receptionist

Secretaries and receptionists must appreciate the situation that when dealing with grieving relatives, sympathy, understanding and patience may be required. They should ensure that the death certificate is available when required, and clearly explain what the relatives/representatives should do with it, for example, taking it to the registrar's office within the statutory time, and, if necessary, give them directions.

Cremation certificates

Doctors may be requested to sign cremation certificates for patients they have attended during their last illness. Cremation certificates require confirmation by another doctor. Two signatures are always necessary, and a doctor may be asked to sign in either capacity. These certificates are available from local funeral directors, and the secretary/receptionist may be asked to ensure that there are forms available when required. A fee is payable to both signatories.

Private certification

Private certificates are issued to patients for purposes outside the scope of the NHS. They are used to supply information to organizations regarding proof of illness, for example:

- holiday insurance

- sick pay and superannuation purposes
- solicitors
- insurance companies
- schools.

A fee may be charged for private certificates. The **BMA** make recommendations of fees, and doctors will charge according to their recommended scale.

Certificate of stillbirth

A doctor must sign a certificate of stillbirth if they were present at the delivery or examined the body of a stillborn child, and give it to the person who will inform the registrar.

Birth registration

Every live or stillbirth must be registered within 42 days. It is the duty of either of the parents to register the birth. In the case of an illegitimate child, the duty to register the birth rests on the mother.

All certificates should either be stamped with the doctor's name, address etc., or may be printed in the case of a private certificate.

The Local Medical Officer must be notified of all births, either by the hospital or the doctor in attendance.

Abortion certificates

The law in Britain allows doctors to terminate pregnancies as long as certain conditions are met:

1   Two doctors must see the patient,
2   They must agree that the conditions laid down in the 1967 Abortion Act have been satisfied.

Note: Conditions allow doctors to recommend termination when they feel that to continue with the pregnancy would be a hazard to either the physical or mental welfare of the pregnant woman or any existing children of her family.

Secretaries and receptionists may be responsible for ensuring the appropriate certification forms are available when required (Figure 4.3).

ABORTION ACT 1967

Not to be destroyed within three years of the date of operation

**Certificate to be completed before an abortion is
performed under Section 1(1) of the Act**

I, ...
(Name and qualifications of practitioner in block capitals)

of ....

....
(Full address of practitioner)

Have/have not* seen/and examined* the pregnant woman to whom this certificate relates at

....

....
(full address of place at which patient was seen or examined)

on ....

and I ....
(Name and qualifications of practitioner in block capitals)

of ....

....
(Full address of practitioner)

Have/have not* seen/and examined* the pregnant woman to whom this certificate relates at

....

....
(Full address of place at which patient was seen or examined)

on ....

We hereby certify that we are of the opinion, formed in good faith, that in the case

of ....
(Full name of pregnant woman in block capitals)

of ....

....
(Usual place of residence of pregnant woman in block capitals)

(Ring appropriate letter(s))	A	the continuance of the pregnancy would involve risk to the life of the pregnant woman greater than if the pregnancy were terminated;
	B	the termination is necessary to prevent grave permanent injury to the physical or mental health of the pregnant woman;
	C	the pregnancy has NOT exceeded its 24th week and that the continuance of the pregnancy would involve risk, greater than if the pregnancy were terminated, of injury to the physical or mental health of the pregnant woman;
	D	the pregnancy has NOT exceeded its 24th week and that the continuance of the pregnancy would involve risk, greater than if the pregnancy were terminated, of injury to the physical or mental health of any existing child(ren) of the family of the pregnant woman;
	E	there is a substantial risk that if the child were born it would suffer from such physical or mental abnormalities as to be seriously handicapped.

This certificate of opinion is given before the commencement of the treatment for the termination of pregnancy to which it refers and relates to the circumstances of the pregnant woman's individual case.

Signed ....   **Date** ....

Signed ....   **Date** ....

* Delete as appropriate   Printed in the U.K. for H.M.S.O. 5/91 Dd. 0H001306 C10000 38806 G3994   Form HSA1 (revised 1991)

Figure 4.3   Abortion certification form (sample).

Health and safety at work

The legislation relating to health and safety at work is complex, and although not directly responsible for workplace standards, medical secretaries and receptionists should be aware of the implications of the Health and Safety at Work Etc. Act (1974) and of their personal responsibilities.

Health and Safety at Work Etc. Act (HASAW) 1974

This Act, passed in 1974, is of direct importance to individuals, whether as managers responsible for the safety of staff immediately under their control, or as a member of the team responsible for the health and safety standards in the surgery, hospital outpatient department or clinic. The Health and Safety at Work Etc. Act is a criminal statute and the Health and Safety Executive (HSE) is the enforcement body. Failure to carry out any duty under the Act is an offence and can lead to prosecution.

The aim of the legislation is to provide and create workplace standards for the reduction of known hazards, provision of a safe working environment for employees and adequate training and supervision given as is necessary to ensure, so far as is reasonably practicable, the health and safety at work of employees. All employers must fulfil this obligation. The term 'reasonably practicable' may be inferred from case law and the advice of HSE inspectors.

HSE inspectors have considerable powers, and may enter premises to enforce the law. Although they do not need to ask permission before doing so, they usually telephone to arrange a visit. Sanctions may be imposed upon those who have unlawfully created or permitted hazards, even where nobody has suffered an accident or ill health.

Employees themselves are obliged to take reasonable care to help in meeting this statutory requirement ('legal duty of care').

Duties of employers and employees

The duties arising from the Health and Safety at Work Etc. Act are not difficult to apply. The legislation requires an employer (including a self-employed person, e.g. a GP) to provide and maintain a safe working environment and it establishes powers and penalties to enforce this. The main aim of the Act is to make both employers and employees conscious of the need for safety in all aspects of their work.

Employers' general duties to staff

The most important duty which every employer should fulfil is 'to ensure as far as is reasonably practicable, the health, safety and welfare at work of all his employees' (HASAW 1974).

Written statement of safety policy

An employer should provide information, training and supervision for staff on health and safety matters. Unless there are fewer than five staff, employers must provide a statement of general policy on health and safety and ensure it is implemented; employees should be consulted on its form and content. The written statement may be included in your employment contract. However, in a medical practice, with fewer than five staff, it is not necessary to give everyone a copy, and the statement can be displayed in a public place.

Safety representatives

Safety representatives are usually appointed if an employer recognizes a trade union, e.g. hospitals, health centres. They have a right to challenge the employer on all health and safety matters.

Duties to others using the hospital or surgery

An employer must ensure the safety of anyone using the premises, including patients, medical and pharmaceutical representatives, visitors, builders, tradesmen and health authority staff.

The Act requires the hospital, surgery or clinic to be run so as to ensure that all users of the premises are safe from risks of personal injury and consideration should be given as to whether there are any potential hazards to elderly or disabled patients.

Notifying accidents and dangerous occurrences

An employer should keep a record of accidents. The HSE should be informed of certain serious accidents occurring to anyone using the premises.

Employees' responsibilities

Staff are required to take reasonable care of their own health and safety on the premises, and of the safety of other users of the premises who may be affected by their actions or omissions, and are expected to co-operate with the employer in carrying out these duties. Although employees' duties technically apply while at work, it would be wise to assume that these also apply throughout the time they are on the premises, for example when preparing coffee or lunch in a staff rest room.

Staff must not interfere with or misuse any health and safety equipment, for example, fire exits, fire extinguishers and warning notices.

Health and safety at work – new regulations

In January 1993 six new sets of health and safety at work regulations came into force. They apply to almost all kinds of work activity in hospitals and general practice. Like the health and safety law, they place duties on employers to protect:

- their employees
- others, including members of the public who may be affected by the work being done.

These new regulations are needed to implement six European Community (EC) directives on health and safety at work. At the same time, they are part of the continuing modernization of UK law, and cover:

- health and safety management
- work equipment safety
- manual handling of loads
- workplace conditions
- personal protective equipment
- display screen equipment.

The new regulations require employers to:

- assess the risk to the health and safety of their employees and anyone else who may be affected by their work in order to identify any necessary preventative and protective measures. Employers with five or more employees should write their risk assessment down
- make arrangements for putting into practice the preventative and protective measures that follow from this risk assessment: they should cover planning, organization control and monitoring and review (i.e. the management of health and safety). Again, any employer with five or more employees must put these arrangements in writing
- carry out health surveillance of employees when appropriate
- appoint a competent person (normally an employee) to help devise and apply the protective steps that the risk assessment shows to be necessary
- set up emergency procedures

- give employees information on health and safety matters
- co-operate on health and safety matters with other employers sharing the same premises (e.g. other health authorities)
- make sure employees have adequate health and safety training and are capable enough at their job to avoid risk
- give whatever health and safety information temporary staff need to meet their specific needs.

These regulations also:

- place duties on all employees to follow health and safety instructions and report danger
- extend current health and safety laws which require employers to consult employees' safety representatives and provide facilities for them.

Provision and use of work equipment

These regulations pull together and tidy up various laws governing equipment used at work. These regulations:

- place general duties on all employers
- list minimum requirements for work equipment to deal with selected hazards which apply across all industries and sectors.

Generally speaking, these regulations make explicit what is already provided for elsewhere in current legislation or in good practice. Organizations that have well-chosen and well-maintained equipment need not do any more. The general duties of these regulations require organizations to:

- take into account the working conditions and hazards in the workplace when choosing equipment
- make sure equipment is suitable for the use intended and that it is properly maintained
- give adequate information, instruction and training.

Manual handling

These regulations replace patchy, old-fashioned and largely ineffective legislation, with a modern ergonomic approach to the problems of manual handling. They are important because the incorrect handling of loads may cause injuries, resulting in pain, time off work and even permanent disablement.

They apply to any manual handling operation which may cause injury at work; these should have been identified by the risk assessment carried out under the general health and safety management regulations described above. They include not only lifting loads, but also lowering, pushing, pulling, carrying or moving them, whether by hand or other bodily force. Again these regulations are supported by general guidance.

There are health care areas where staff are at risk in this respect, for example, nursing.

Employers have to take three key steps.

1   Avoid hazardous manual handling operations when reasonably practicable.
2   Assess adequately any hazardous operations that cannot be avoided.
3   Reduce the risk of injury as far as possible.

Workforce health, safety and welfare

These regulations tidy up a lot of existing legislation, replacing some 35 pieces of old law. They are much easier to understand and make it far clearer what is expected. They cover many aspects of health, safety and welfare in the workplace, setting general requirements in four broad areas:

1   *Working environment* – temperature, ventilation, lighting, room dimensions, suitability of work stations.
2   *Safety* – safe passage of pedestrians and vehicles, windows and skylights (safe opening, closing and cleaning), safe materials and marking for transparent doors and partitions, doors, gates and escalators (safety devices), safe doors, gates and escalators, floors, falls from heights and falling objects.
3   *Facilities* – toilets, washing, eating and changing facilities, clothing storage, seating, rest areas, arrangements for non-smokers, rest facilities for pregnant women and nursing mothers.
4   *Housekeeping* – maintenance of workplace, equipment and facilities, cleanliness, and removal of waste materials.

Employers should ensure premises comply with the regulations but this does not have to be completed until 1996 for existing premises.

Personal protective equipment

These regulations set out sound principles for selecting, providing, maintaining and using personal protective equipment (PPE). They are not directly relevant to medical secretaries and receptionists so further information would appear inappropriate.

Display screen equipment (DSE)

Unlike most of the regulations previously listed, the health and safety (display screen equipment) regulations do not replace old legislation, but cover a new area of work activity. Working with DSE is not generally risky, but it can lead to musculoskeletal problems, eye fatigue and mental stress. Problems of this kind can be overcome by good ergonomic design of equipment, furniture, the working environment and the tasks performed.

The regulations apply to DSE where there is a 'user', i.e. an employee who habitually uses it as a significant part of normal work. They cover equipment used for the display of text, numbers and graphics, regardless of the display process used.

These regulations include:

- assessing DSE workstations and reducing risks which are identified

- making sure workstations satisfy minimum requirements set for the DSE itself – keyboard, desk and chair, working environment and task design and software

- planning DSE work, so that there are breaks or changes in inactivity

- providing information and training for DSE users.

DSE users are entitled to appropriate eye and eyesight tests, and to special glasses if they are needed and normal ones cannot be used. Again these regulations are supported by detailed guidelines which are contained in the Health and Safety Executive's Guidance Note on DSE Work.

The Control of Substances Hazardous to Health Regulations (COSHH) 1988

COSHH regulations set out guidelines for the control of hazardous substances to employers, who have an obligation to protect people exposed to such substances.

The regulations include virtually all substances which are hazardous to health, and clearly sets out the essential measures which employers, self-employed, and sometimes employees, have to take. Failure to comply constitutes an offence under the Health and Safety at Work Etc. Act. Substances hazardous to health include those labelled as:

- dangerous

- toxic

- harmful

- irritant

- corrosive.

The regulations give guidelines to employers which are based upon principles of occupational hygiene, the key duties being:

- to identify substances hazardous to health in the workplace

- to formally assess (in writing) the risk to employees from these materials

- to control adequately and monitor the risk

- to provide health surveillance where appropriate

- to provide adequate instruction and training.

Other less dangerous substances covered by the regulations include disinfectants, clinical wastes, cleaning materials and, of course, drugs.

GPs, health authorities and other health care employers should consider how COSHH applies to the working environment and to their employees, for example:

- the risk from biocides and sterilizing agents

- the risk of staff contracting infection from biological samples and waste

- policies and specific procedures are necessary for cleaning medical equipment, and safe disposal of drugs, contaminated needles, dressings and appliances

- staff vaccination status should be reviewed.

Summary of legal aspects

This section has attempted to give an overview of the many and diverse legal aspects involving the work of medical secretaries and receptionists.

On a more personal note, information has been given to provide a basic knowledge and understanding of legislation influencing the duties and rights of employees and employers working in organizations, large or small.

5

Health and safety in a clinical environment

Introduction

General principles of health and safety at work have already been discussed in some detail. On a practical issue, how does it affect the secretary and receptionist working in a clinical environment?

The Health and Safety at Work Etc. Act requires:

- *That any 'plant' in the workplace is safe* – The term plant covers equipment in the practice, including heaters, sterilizers, electric kettles, plugs and examination couches.

  Potential hazards include someone getting a shock from an electric kettle due to a plug incorrectly fitted; tripping over a cable trailing across the room; a patient being injured because an examination couch collapses. Occurrences such as these could lead to a charge of having unsafe plant on the premises and ensuing liability.

- *That systems of work are safe* – It is important that the day-to-day running of the practice does not lead to injury, for example, lifting heavy boxes from the floor causing back strain could be considered as 'unsafe'. Also, careless handling of pathological specimens or patients hurting themselves on prams and bicycles left outside the surgery, may be considered as unsafe working practice.

- *That premises are safe* – This includes floors which are slippery or dangerous when wet, outside steps which are unlit at night, and ceilings in danger of collapse, which could all be considered as unsafe.

First aid at work

Regulations require employers to make adequate provision for their employees in case of injury or if they should become unwell at work. There is no need for a trained first-aider, but there must be an appointed person available at all times. This person is to take charge of the situation if a serious injury or illness occurs in the absence of medical or nursing staff. They are responsible for the first-aid equipment. An 'appointed' person should have attended a short course in first aid lasting at least four hours, which should include:

- resuscitation

- control of bleeding

- treatment of the unconscious casualty.

Hazardous substances in the workplace

Control of Substances Hazardous to Health (COSHH) regulations have already been mentioned. Receptionists and secretaries should be aware of hazards arising from the handling, transport and disposal of hazardous substances, not only for their own protection but to ensure that their place of work is not in breach of the law.

Clinical waste

Clinical waste is waste arising from medical practice that may provide a hazard or give offence unless rendered safe and inoffensive. Such waste includes human or animal tissue, or excretion, drugs and medicinal products, swabs, dressings, instruments or similar substances and materials.

All staff involved in areas where clinical waste arises should be given instruction in waste handling, segregation, storage and disposal procedures, and where appropriate, the use of protective clothing.

Waste segregation

This is achieved by readily identifiable colour-coded containers:

- *Black* – Normal household waste, not to be used for clinical waste

- *Yellow* – All waste to be incinerated.

There are different categories of waste and different procedures for each category. These include:

- soiled surgical dressings, swabs and other contaminated waste from consulting rooms and treatment areas
- syringes, needles, cartridges and glass ampoules ('sharps')
- laboratory waste in medical practice, includes blood samples after testing, vomit or sputum
- solid dose medicinal products, small volume injectables, vaccine and sera*
- urine samples.

Secretaries and receptionists will be given appropriate instructions for disposal if necessary. However, the following guidelines should be understood by all those working in medical practice.

Storage of clinical waste

Waste bags must be kept secure from unauthorized persons and entry by animals whilst awaiting collection. They must never be left outside where children may play, or drug addicts may find used syringes and needles.

Removal of clinical waste

This is arranged on a local basis. Health authorities/health boards will advise on the availability of a collection service. Organizations providing this service will arrange to supply waste disposal and arrange collection and incineration.

Specimens

Handling specimens

Receptionists in general practice may find that patients leave various specimens on the reception counter unwrapped. It is the receptionist's duty to protect herself and colleagues from potential infection by handling these specimens correctly, for example either ask the patient to place the specimen in a plastic bag, or use a pair of disposable gloves to handle the specimen. The same system could be used for handling used medicine containers, dressings, tissues, hearing aids, etc.

* *Note:* All controlled drugs covered by the Misuse of Drugs Act require special procedures before they can be destroyed.

Transport of specimens

Specimens to be sent to the pathology laboratory by the local collection service must be clearly labelled and accompanied by pathology request forms. Specimens to be sent by post must be packaged in a rigid container with absorbent packing and sent by first-class letter post. The address of the sender should be clearly written on the outside of the package so that the post office can contact the sender if the package is damaged to find out the risk to the handler. Specimens sent through the post must be clearly labelled 'Pathological Specimen–Handle with Care'.

Hepatitis and AIDS

Receptionists are at risk where blood, semen, and other body fluids of an infected person can enter the body, for example, through an open cut. All scratches, cuts and grazes must be covered with a waterproof covering.

When body fluid has to be mopped up, disposable plastic or latex gloves, a disposable plastic apron and paper tissues must be used *whether or not* infection is present. After use, these items must be placed in a waste collection unit for incineration. Clothing may be cleaned by washing on a hot-cycle. Hard surfaces and floors can be wiped/washed with a freshly prepared 10% bleach solution. Skin that has been in contact should be washed with soap and water. Mouth-to-mouth resuscitation should be carried out with a mouthpiece if available. Common sense measures and good hygiene are the best measures to prevent infection.

Fire Precautions Act (1971)

This is the Act covering fire regulations. However, in medical practices with less than 20 people working, there is no need for a fire certificate. Larger organizations, e.g. hospitals and health centres will have regular fire drills. The local fire officer will check the provision of fire alarms, extinguishers and hoses, that fire exits are not obstructed and signs are readily visible. Provision of emergency light supplies are checked.

Medical practices should have their own plans and clearly defined procedures to be followed in the event of fire. Basic guidelines would include:

- prevention – check for hazards and try to prevent a fire from happening

- fire alert/warning – who will raise the alarm and dial 999? Who will evacuate the surgery? What is the system for ensuring that everyone in the building knows about it? How to stop more patients from entering

- evacuation – procedures for evacuating the building. Marshall all staff and patients to one assembly point. How do you ensure no one is missing?

- security – people are most important. Leave behind all valuables, except the appointment book which will tell you if anyone is missing. This should be taken to the assembly point

- informing staff and public – a notice should be displayed telling people what to do in the event of fire. The notice should indicate the placing of fire extinguishers and exits.

Coping with aggression and violence

Dealing with aggressive callers

Receptionists and secretaries working in the field of health care face a number of patients and callers who are potentially violent, for example, the mentally disturbed, the emotionally upset, or those who are suffering from the effects of drugs or drink.

Your organization will, no doubt, have a policy for dealing with potentially violent patients. If so, it is up to you to ensure you know what it is and what you should do. Remember, most of the patients attending your hospital or your surgery are seeking understanding, help and advice about their problems which are causing them a certain amount of anxiety. They may become frustrated and aggrieved as they wait for their appointments.

As the patient becomes more upset, it can lead to aggression and the receptionist or secretary may be the focus of this aggression. Always deal as quickly as possible with any patient who becomes agitated, especially if they seem to be under the influence of drugs or drink. Make sure you alert the doctor or nurse to the problem as soon as possible.

When a confrontation is building up, try to defuse the situation by talking to the patient in a calm manner, and attempt to reduce that patient's agitation. You may be able to distract the patient from his/her particular grievance and cool the situation.

You should be on guard to protect yourself from physical attack. In trying to appear relaxed and natural you may, for example, put your hands in your pockets; this will leave you defenceless to a blow. If possible, always get a physical barrier between you and the aggressor, such as a counter or a desk. Discreetly try to attract the attention of another member of staff if it seems as if the situation is going to erupt. If you have a buzzer 'alert' system, have a pre-arranged signal and use it.

Note: The best way to defend yourself from attack is to get out of the way as quickly as possible.

Coping with a personal attack

A personal attack is unlikely to happen, and if you take commonsense precautions you can reduce the risk. Unfortunately, some attacks do occur and you should give some thought about what you should do if you become a victim.

Always remember that personal safety should come before property. Is it worth being injured for the sake of a prescription or some tablets? The police would prefer you uninjured and in a position to give them an accurate description of the attacker.

It is worth considering what you would be prepared to do in self defence should you be attacked. If other people are near, then you must shout to attract their attention. Only you can decide whether to fight back. A woman has the right to defensive action using reasonable force in the case of an attack, for example, by kicking, scratching or by the use of items which are accepted as normally being carried:

- hair spray

- bunch of keys

- umbrella

- personal attack alarm.

It must be pointed out, however, that legally you may not carry offensive weapons.

If you are sexually assaulted or raped, it is important that you contact the police immediately – for your own sake and for the safety of others. Always bear in mind:

- however difficult or unpleasant the thought, resist the need to wash or change your clothing – you could be removing important evidence

- do not drink alcohol or take any drugs that might prevent you from giving a clear account of what has happened

- try to remember as much as possible about your attacker.

The police will deal with you with care, understanding and complete confidentiality.

General security and safety in the surgery or hospital

- Challenge all suspicious persons.

- Do not be taken in by so-called workmen or officials; if they are genuine, they will not mind having their identity checked.

- Keep all valuables and prescription pads out of sight.

- Ensure petty cash is secured in a locked tin, and kept inside a locked drawer.

- Ensure consulting and treatment rooms are locked when not in use.

- If you have an identity badge, always wear it.

- Equipment should be security marked.

- Always keep your valuables with you, or lock them away.

Travelling to and from work or whenever you are out and about

You should always be alert to potential danger when travelling by car, public transport or on foot. Remember the following points:

- think ahead. Get into a safe routine and always use it

- avoid walking home late at night

- walk purposefully. Do *not* accept lifts

- when travelling by car, do not give lifts to strangers

- on public transport sit near the guard, driver or other women passengers

- only use a reputable taxi cab firm. Ask the cab company for the driver's name and call sign

- in the event of your car breaking down and waiting for help, keep doors and windows locked and sit in the passenger seat so it appears you are not alone

- avoid multi-storey car parks where possible

- carry a torch with you if travelling after dark.

Safety at the end of a surgery or clinic session

Always check that the premises are secure before you leave, and look outside to make sure that no one is lurking. If you see someone prowling or hanging around, stay inside and let someone know. If necessary, contact the police. If you are usually collected by car, wait until it arrives before going out. If you are travelling by public transport and are alone, do not leave so early that you have to wait a long time for the bus or train.

Finally, your local crime prevention officer attached to your nearest police station will be willing to talk to you and your colleagues about coping with aggression and violence and give practical help and advice to women on their personal safety.

6

Practical reception skills in general practice

Introduction

Every receptionist is gifted in some way, for example in dealing kindly with people, having patience, a pleasant speaking voice, etc. In addition to these natural gifts everyone can acquire skills to help them to do their job better. The most important skill areas are those of communication and organization which are covered in other areas of this text. However, there are some skills which are unique to a receptionist in general practice.

All approaches to the receptionist are by patients, or their relatives, who believe that they have a need. They cannot see 'behind the scenes' in the surgery or have any real understanding of the pressures on doctors and receptionists. Receptionists must always bear in mind the perceived need of the patient, no matter how insignificant from the surgery perspective. Patients are concerned about either their own state of health or that of a family member. It is very important, therefore, that the skills to recognize how patients are feeling and deal sensitively with them are used constantly. The issues of non-verbal communication and related issues are covered in Chapter 2.

The person responsible for controlling the flow of patients into a number of doctors consulting at the same time needs to have a good system, to concentrate and remain alert. If other members are fully co-operative in matters like ensuring the appointments book, or surgery lists, are clearly written, or appropriately 'marking off' a patient as arriving, or having been sent into the doctor, then the task is made simpler. However, the person controlling the surgery flow tends to be the one to whom everyone turns with queries - Where are Mrs A's results? Where are the notes for child B? Do I need to do a claim form for child health surveillance? How many extras are there? When will Dr C be free to see the rep? and so on. If telephone answering also is part of the picture, it can be very difficult to keep on top of who is where, and what needs to be dealt with next.

Smooth surgery flow is made easier if the preparation for surgeries has been carried out properly. Where an appointment system is used it is sensible to take out all the medical records well before the start of surgery and check that all test results and hospital letters relating to these records have been filed. It can also help the practice finances if stickers are used on the records to indicate that smears are due or pill forms need to be signed, which the receptionist can then act upon by drawing the doctor's attention with a note, or completing a claim ready for signature.

As patients leave the consulting room follow-up appointments need to be arranged, and appropriate advice given about requirements for some health promotion clinics, e.g. to bring a urine sample. Maintaining neat work areas during consulting times makes tidying at the end of surgery considerably easier. However, even if it is not possible to keep tidy at the busiest times it is important that quieter times are used to the fullest to return working areas to order, file medical records, check that doctors' rooms have been tidied and stocks of disposables topped up.

Telephone answering can be an especially difficult task for the doctor's receptionist. Any incoming call may be about a patient who is bleeding, appearing to have a heart attack, or some other medical crisis with a child. Therefore, the procedure for dealing with emergencies must be clear and the telephone must never be left to ring for an indefinite period. The telephone must be answered in preference to dealing with a patient standing at the reception desk – however, it is also essential that any patient at the desk is acknowledged with a smile, so that they know they will be dealt with when you are free.

The receptionist is also required to be a fount of all knowledge, for example, the following can be helpful in finding and giving out appropriate information efficiently:

- keeping telephone directories of often-used numbers, or hospital internal directories, along with other service information sources

- list of subjects of leaflets kept available for patients in the waiting room and brief notes on developments in trends in health promotion

- awareness of changes to surgeries and clinics, changes in local hospital, community and social services.

It is especially important that the receptionist knows the limits of her own authority, i.e. when and to whom to refer for advice.

The receptionist is also responsible for keeping an eye on the waiting area to:

- make sure that the patients who are obviously unwell are not troubled by unduly active children

- maintain a pleasant ambience, by ensuring adequate ventilation or heat

- tidy the waiting area of toys, magazines and leaflets at the end of each surgery or clinic.

Thankfully, it will rarely be necessary to clean up whilst patients are waiting, for example, if a patient is literally sick in the waiting area or walks something unpleasant-smelling from the pavement into the surgery!

Keeping the doctors happy is yet another set of tasks for the receptionist. Most of the time this will entail keeping the surgery flow steady, not allowing too many interruptions in consultations, providing tea or coffee at the right times, and making sure that records, results, letters and other essentials are all available when required. Not too much to ask!

Individually controlling surgery flow, answering the telephone, dealing with patients at the desk, and keeping the doctor happy are not too difficult to achieve as separate items, but in the real world of the reception office, there is rarely the opportunity to concentrate on one task at a time. The skill is in being able to constantly readjust priorities, without forgetting the ones that slip to the bottom of the mental pile.

Dividing up the duties so that, for instance, one person controls surgery flow, another majors on answering the telephone, another does repeat scripts and perhaps deals with queries, can go some way to lessening the pressure. However, it is also impossible to remain rigidly with such a plan. It is essential that receptionists work in a team, not only being aware of keeping on top of what they are supposed to be doing, but having their eyes open to see when a colleague needs help, and being able to adjust their own priorities to step into the breach.

Various tools, like log books, message books, having good systems in place, clear procedures for dealing with routine issues, knowing whom to turn to with queries, all help. However, the ability to juggle ten priorities at one time is both an art and a gift. Being self-controlled, planning work, and being as efficient about it as possible means that anyone with a degree of intelligence, who wants to, can achieve a certain degree of competency. However, there will always be some people who enjoy this kind of pressure (only feeling the strain sometimes) and those to whom it is a strain all the time.

First impressions

First impressions count. A receptionist will often be the patient's initial point of contact with the organization, and they will make assumptions, positive or negative, about the treatment they are likely to receive from that first point.

Record keeping and general administration

In any business it is essential to keep records. For example, where a receptionist may be delegated the task of keeping control of stocks of forms and stationery, or petty cash it is essential that adequate documentation is maintained. Alternatively a receptionist is likely to pass messages to a variety of people in the course of a working day. Keeping a record of messages ensures that not only does the right message get passed, but who took the message, who received it and when, can all be substantiated.

Written communication

Although technology is coming on apace there is still the need for hand-written communication – messages and notes to one another. It is obvious that any hand-written communication should be legible, but often in haste it is easy to forget that, and to fail to ensure that any other person should be able to read a scrawled message, entry in an appointment book or list of names, etc.

Messages

Some offices have pre-printed message forms which prompt message takers to collect all the necessary information as they go. Another option is to use a message book with columns drawn up, so that it is easy to check if a message has been received. It is important not only that there should be adequate systems for communicating messages, but responsibility is taken to ensure that the systems work properly.

Message boards

Dry-wipe white boards are extremely useful for putting up short-term reminders and messages, provided one person is delegated responsibility for clearing off messages as soon as they become redundant!

Letters, memos and report writing

Receptionists may be required to send out letters, memos and generate reports. As a general rule this is likely to be routine (standard) documents, where a master copy is used to generate photocopies, into which names and addresses, dates, data, can be inserted by hand. However, technology has made it possible for receptionists with little or no formal training in secretarial or wordprocessing skills to generate printed letters from the computer. It is important to remember that the image of the practice/hospital is presented via written communication and therefore it is important that presentation standards are met. There are conventions about letter layout, e.g., whether commas are used at the end of every line in an address or how many spaces are left between the end of a letter and 'Yours sincerely'. Where training is not given in these details a poor impression will be given to anyone who expects normal conventions to be observed. Therefore, the setting of practice standards is a valuable guide to ensure that everyone produces written communication to the same standard.

Organization

Systems and organization are essential to the smooth running of a reception area. Some are blessed with a natural ability to be organized. Those who are not need to apply far more self-discipline to initiate and maintain systems. Everyone needs to know what is expected of whom, using what, and by when.

Similarly, individuals need to be organized in their use of time. The receptionist who retains control of the tasks to be completed avoids personal stress. Too much stress will inevitably lead to mistakes, poor handling of patients, and a general deterioration in standards of service.

Take time out to:

- make a list of the tasks you perform every day, every week, once a month

– make a week plan

– block off the times on the week plan you have no option but to be 'demand driven', e.g. on reception desk for a busy surgery/clinic

– fit other tasks around these blocks at the optimum time

- make a 'to do' list

– break down big items into small stages

– realistically allocate items from your 'to do' list into your working week

- discuss your findings with your supervisor so that any queries regarding priorities can be settled to their satisfaction.

Using the simple example of stocks of forms, unless there is a system for ensuring that stocks are maintained there is every likelihood that either one day stores will run out or that scarce storage space is taken up by unnecessarily large supplies.

Since there are many supplies needed it is helpful if a system is set up and maintained with the same degree of commitment from everyone.

Initial skill is needed to think through the best and simplest way of organizing any particular aspect of reception, after that, discipline and commitment from all team members are essential to maintain the system.

Maintaining the office and reception areas

In order to ensure the comfort and well being of patients, relatives and other visitors, effort needs to be made to keep public areas tidy and smart. This must be a priority, because untidiness can be a hazard and gives a general impression of sloppiness.

Ensure that:

- the area is kept tidy and free from hazards. Some visitors are likely to have visual or physical disabilities

- hazards are reported promptly and immediate action taken to minimize the danger

- fire exits are clearly indicated and kept unobstructed

- notices and information leaflets are kept up to date, and are clearly and neatly displayed

- an up-to-date supply of magazines, etc., is available for visitors to read.

Mail

Mail should be correctly sorted and date stamped on receipt. Any enclosures should be securely attached and missing items reported promptly. The mail should then be passed to the appropriate person for action.

When sending mail out check that names and addresses are correct and clearly legible. Envelopes and parcels should be securely sealed. All the mail you deal with should be handled promptly as it relates to patients' health and any delay could be dangerous.

If you are suspicious of any mail received, local security arrangements should be followed. Check with your manager if you are unfamiliar with these.

Stock control

The purpose of stock control system is to keep track of such items as sta-tionery, computer hardware, drugs, dressings, linen, sundry equipment, etc. that the practice possesses. A stock control system is necessary to avoid two pitfalls:

1   *Having too much stock.* Money tied up in stock cannot be used for any other purpose, and if the stock is perishable or becomes obsolete as time passes, it may be difficult to recover this money in full.
2   *Having too little stock.* If essential items are short, patients may face long delays or inconvenience.

The ideal situation, and the one that a good stock control system aims to produce, is to have adequate stock on hand – neither too much nor too little.

Stock control also acts as a deterrent to wastage and pilfering. A good system will show up when losses are occurring, and the knowledge of this may deter pilferers. It should also highlight the points at which losses are likely to occur from other causes.

Records of stock levels are obviously essential to any large-scale control system; a hospital which does not keep control of stocks is likely to find it very hard to control them efficiently. The records may be on index cards, or a computerized stock control system may be in operation. Goods are stored until they are needed, and are released by the storekeeper only when he or she is presented with a duly authorized document, such as a requisition note.

Petty cash

Small amounts of expenditure for goods or services are usually paid for out of petty cash since the amounts are too small to be paid by cheque, for example, stamps, milk bills, small stationery items. Secretarial or clerical staff may be responsible for controlling petty cash and the system most commonly used is known as the *imprest* system.

The imprest amount is drawn from the account each week or month, through the main cash book. The sum is estimated to cover all small expenses throughout the agreed period, and is referred to as the 'imprest' or 'float'. The petty cash is kept in a locked cash box. During the month, payments are made from the imprest, and all expenditure must be covered by a petty cash voucher or a receipt. The voucher should be signed by the person receiving the money. The vouchers and receipts should be num-bered and filed for purposes of audit.

A separate petty cash book is maintained analysing the expenditure, and at the end of the month a sum of money is drawn by cheque to restore the amount of the imprest to the original sum.

Helping to maintain a safe environment

Health and safety at work legislation is intended to safeguard all employees, patients and visitors to the workplace. Individual employees are required to ensure that they do not endanger their own health or safety, or that of their colleagues, patients or visitors. Potentially dangerous situations and unknown or potentially hazardous substances must be treated with the utmost care.

The legislation is detailed and complex. As a minimum, all staff must ensure that:

- there are no trailing wires
- filing cabinet drawers are kept closed
- chairs and other obstacles do not block walkways or fire escapes
- fire extinguishers and exits are clearly indicated
- any known hazards are marked clearly and problems reported to the appropriate manager
- visitors are informed of any known hazards
- potentially violent situations are defused as far as is possible
- care is taken when handling specimens, especially over spillages, and hands are washed after undertaking this task.

Coping with aggression and violence

Communication is often the key when dealing with conflict of this kind. Good communication can play a vital part in defusing potentially difficult situations or avoiding them altogether, but equally, poor communication can increase levels of frustration and anger which then erupt in violence. We have to consider carefully what messages our words and movements are conveying. Are they contradictory? We can tell when someone is saying one thing but means something quite different. Perhaps it is someone we know well, and can therefore judge their statements on the basis of what we know of them, but it is equally likely that they are strangers, and the truth is conveyed by their stance, facial movements, etc. (see Chapter 5).

Procedures manuals

Many organizations are using Standard Operating Procedures (SOPs) as part of implementing BS5750. These SOPs state who does what, how they should do it, how often, etc.

Within reception offices there may not be the need to have SOPs for every activity or task, but a manual of key procedures may be helpful. The administrative processes of stock control and petty cash are two examples which should be documented in a specific procedure. The procedure document may be as little as one side of A4 with the vital information summarized into a table, but it should include who is responsible, what steps are taken, how frequently, and any special notes. Filing these procedure sheets into a loose-leaf folder allows additional procedures to be added or existing procedures to be updated whenever necessary. Apart from encouraging a uniform approach to carrying out tasks, these written procedures form a useful resource especially for new staff who may have been told how to do something, but have forgotten or need to clarify details.

Information technology (IT)

Practices still vary enormously in their modes of working, in size, number of staff, equipment available, and capability of using their technology.

Computer

Where a practice has the patient database on computer the advantages include:

- logging and generation of repeat prescriptions
- checking registration status
- checking immunization/smear status
- checking health promotion data.

If this is linked into an appointments system the difficulties of manual appointment books, e.g. illegible writing, pages messy with cancellations, two people not being able to use the book at the same time, hand-written surgery lists for pulling out records, are all circumvented.

The major disadvantage is when the system 'goes down', all this increased efficiency disappears and returning to manual methods, no matter how temporarily, results in unavoidable delays and disruption.

Reference has been made to IT for written communication in Chapter 10. Suffice to say here that staff who could only ever write letters are now able to use wordprocessing to generate mailmerged letters, or produce their own letters to patients with very little training. Spreadsheets can be used either to collect data (for display in tables, graphs and pie charts) or to present doctor and staff rotas.

Desk-top publishing software can be used to generate leaflets, posters and handouts. Technology saves time for some tasks: in others it does not save time, but it does make it possible to produce professional-looking documents, e.g. rota charts, posters.

For those who enjoy using the computer it is essential that the computer does not become an obstacle between the patient and the receptionist. It is equally rude to continue to type away absorbed by the machine as it is to continue to talk to a colleague or take a telephone call without acknowledging the presence of a patient.

The advantage of technology to receptionists include:

- ease of presenting professional standard documents, speed of finding, generating and transmitting information
- efficiency in dealing with issues.

The major disadvantages to receptionists include:

- reliance upon the electronics so that in the event of the computer 'being down' everything has to go on hold
- the danger of losing the personal touch.

Fax and electronic mail

The fax machine has several important uses in general practice:

- to return urgent blood results
- notification of discharge from maternity wards
- to pass complex information
- make claims to FHSA, health boards/registrations, etc.

In general the advantages and disadvantages to the receptionist using the fax machine may be summarized:

ADVANTAGES	DISADVANTAGES
Cheaper than using the telephone (if it takes less time to say it)	Breach of confidentiality if fax goes to the wrong address
Much quicker than the post	Fax paper may fade with time, so it is important either to photocopy or file the original

Photocopying

The photocopier is a great time saver. However, lack of training in office standards and procedures can result in poor quality work and failure to maintain the equipment properly. Good quality originals are essential to producing fine quality copies. A ring binder can be kept near to the photocopier with photocopy originals in clear plastic wallets. (Yellow highlighter pen does not show up on the photocopies, so use one to write 'original' to ensure that the original is easily identifiable and does not get circulated.)

Costs can be kept down by reducing the number of poor quality copies by simple things such as:

- collecting a folder of good quality 'originals'

- ensuring that the original does not get used

- placing the original carefully, so that copies do not come out even slightly skew

- buying appropriate cleaners

- never putting documents with wet correction fluid onto the platen

- keeping the platen (the glass panel onto which copies are placed) clean

- delegating someone to be responsible for replacing the toner and keeping the copier clean.

The effect of technology on staff is to make their lives a lot easier in some ways, and to make aspects of work available to them for personal development, the disadvantage for people who are afraid of technology is that they may get left behind and their value falls because they cannot take an equal share in routine workloads.

A receptionist is now required to have a wide range of skills. Apart from dealing with people on the telephone and face to face, retrieving and filing medical records and filing away letters and reports, the receptionist generally needs to have keyboard skills and a willingness to learn how to use the latest technology.

Appointment systems in general practice

The role that the medical receptionist plays is crucial to the successful running of an appointment system. Nearly every patient who sees the doctor makes his or her first contact through the receptionist. The receptionist channels patients into the appointment system and runs the system once the surgery has started.

The receptionist has to calm the agitated patient, explain and cope with doctors' absences on emergencies, and acts to translate unstreamed demand into a rational framework.

It is important to run an appointment system as well as possible, both for the doctor and the patient's sake – even a few dissatisfied patients can lead very quickly to an unhappy practice. A well run system reflects the general efficiency of the practice, and puts less strain on GPs and their receptionists.

An efficient appointment system should benefit both doctor and patient:

Benefits to doctors

- effective organization of workload
- more efficient management of time
- limits the number of patients seen in one session
- patients records are left on their desks in advance of surgery session
- less waiting room space required
- the duration of consultation can be varied according to predetermined need

Benefits to patients

- able to plan their day
- should not have to wait a long time to see the doctor
- fewer people in the waiting room – less chance of cross-infection.

The perfect appointment system is neither too rigid to exclude emergencies, nor so chaotic that it keeps those who have made appointments waiting for an excessive length of time. The number of patients booked for each surgery session should bear a close relation to the speed at which the doctor works.

Patient dissatisfaction arises from not being able to get an appointment without delay. Appointment systems, therefore, should be flexible to allow for those patients with urgent problems to see their doctor very quickly.

The terms 'urgent' and 'emergency' are both subjective and emotive terms, and perhaps receptionists should be encouraged to delete them from their vocabulary! They could be replaced with 'will it wait until tomorrow?' However, your practice will have its own procedures for dealing with such requests from patients.

Types of appointment system

Times of booking for patients can be arranged in various ways and each practice or doctor will decide which system suits them best.

Whatever system is used, it is essential for the frequency of appointments to match the doctor's consultation rate, and for sufficient time to be left for patients who need to be seen and fitted in at short notice.

Your surgery may use one or a combination of the following types of booking:

- sequential booking

- block-release booking

- limited block booking.

All these systems have the flexibility for patients to be seen quickly if necessary. There are several ways to deal with 'extras' to be seen despite a full appointments book:

- they can be fitted in between booked appointments

- provision can be made for patients with urgent problems to be seen after the booked surgery

- one doctor in the practice on a rotating basis, to act as 'mopper-up' and see the extras instead of carrying out a booked surgery

- block-release booking allows for 'holes' to be left in the appointments book which cannot be filled until the beginning of the day on which they are entered

Whichever method your practice uses, it is essential that the receptionist knows exactly what to do.

Follow-up after missed appointments

Patients who fail to keep their appointments for cervical cytology and immunizations will either be sent a letter or telephoned with a further appointment. If patients do not attend, doctors may not achieve their targets for cervical cytology and child immunization.

The medical records of non-attendees for routine appointments may be marked 'DNA' – 'did not attend' and this information may also be entered on the practice computer. However, this procedure may vary according to practice protocol.

If the doctor has given the patient advice about follow-up appointments, tests, etc. it is important to check their understanding of the instructions given. They may need to be given a letter, or appointment card with the details of their next appointment. If a patient seems to be confused about what has been said, it is doubly important to encourage them to wait and have a word with the doctor or nurse before they leave. The patient may need to be directed to the correct place for any tests which are necessary. After the appointment, the notes will go to the secretary for any letters that are needed.

Medical records

A medical record is the history of a patient's treatment as an outpatient, inpatient or both. The record is vital because it provides a means of communication between doctors, nurses and other members of the care team, about investigations, diagnosis, observations, treatment prescribed, and progress. It acts as a reminder, and can be used as an educational instrument for trainees, for research, for informing medical negligence cases and other legal purposes, and for gathering statistics such as those that are needed for planning future services.

Records contain much confidential information, and all those with access to them have a legal responsibility to maintain confidentiality. Computerized records present a particular challenge to confidentiality. This is examined in more detail in Chapter 7.

Two recent Acts of Parliament allow individuals access to their medical information. The Access to Medical Reports Act 1988 gives an individual in England, Wales or Scotland the right to see medical reports prepared for insurance or employment purposes. The Access to Personal Files and Medical Reports Order 1991 for Northern Ireland affords similar rights there. The Access to Health Records Act 1990, which applies in England, Wales and Scotland, establishes an individual's right of access to their own medical records. In certain circumstances, access can be granted to other individuals. The Act also provides for the correction of inaccurate information. Access can be refused in certain cases if, in the opinion of the record holder, disclosure would cause serious harm to the patient. (See Chapter 4.)

Medical records were standardized when the NHS began to provide some uniformity between hospitals, although some local variation still exists.

In the United Kingdom, the medical records held by general practitioners are unique; they follow patients throughout their lives from the cradle to the grave. Medical records show patients' names, demographic details, and information of previous illnesses and significant episodes in the lives of their subjects, unlike hospital records which often only cover a specific episode of hospital attendance, e.g. appendicitis or hysterectomy.

The purpose of the medical record

The basic function of the medical record can best be described as an 'aide-memoire' (Figure 6.1):

- It gives a method of recording events in a person's life. It traces from birth the record of a patient's illnesses, treatments, investigations and other significant events.

- It is a channel of communication. The GP writes in the medical record, giving details of his/her findings, treatment and diagnosis of a patient's condition. This becomes a permanent record and communicates that information to those persons who have the right of access, for example, another partner in the practice, the practice nurse, or to another doctor at a later date.

- It acts as a record of outside health contacts. When the patient attends a hospital outpatient department, or has an investigation, information is provided, and if correctly filled in, the patient's record contributes to the total knowledge about the patient.

- It provides a record of all treatment and all the drugs given during a patient's lifetime.

- It is a medico-legal record. If a medical or legal problem arises at any time, the patient's medical records will be required to support any action taken.

THE FOUR MAIN FUNCTIONS OF MEDICAL RECORDS

A permanent record of significant events

A medico-legal record

A file for hospital and laboratory reports and letters

An aide-memoire

Thus, it is vital that medical records are kept securely and the information contained therein stored in an orderly, systematic way. This can be achieved by:

- ensuring that all the continuation sheets are in chronological order, starting hopefully from birth, and fixing them in a permanent way, e.g. with a treasury tag, so that new continuation cards can be easily added

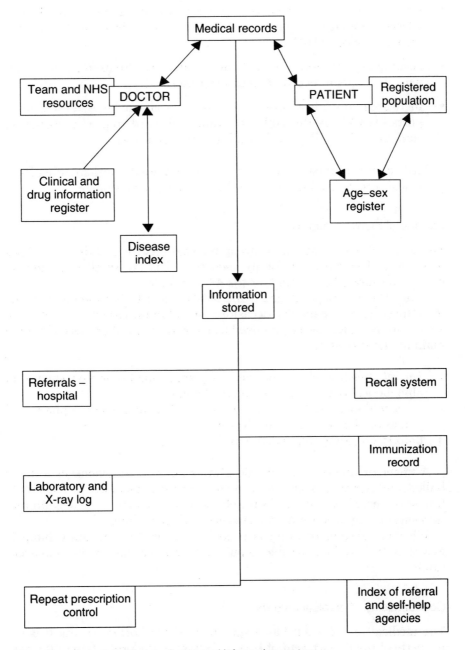

Figure 6.1   A model of the medical record information system.

- keeping hospital records, copies of GPs' letters and any other correspondence in chronological order and fastened together
- dealing with the results of any investigations in the same way
- keeping a summary sheet where the major and significant diseases or allergies are entered. This should be kept in the front of the medical record envelope (MRE)
- keeping prescription summary cards which are also useful as a permanent, easily seen record of all drugs prescribed
- there are many other forms of record card that can be used for specific purpose, such as the child immunization card, repeat prescription summary, obstetric record, contraceptive record, etc.

Medical receptionists and secretaries should not discard anything from a medical record envelope without the doctor's permission.

Storage of medical records

There are different ways of grouping medical records and different types of records. The most commonly used record is the small size medical record envelope (7in. x 5½in.), or the A4-size folder.

Some practices separate male and female records, but the majority file them together. There may be occasions when families are filed together in an A4 family folder. Every practice has its own system, but there are three main methods of storage:

1 *Lateral* shelving where records are placed side-by-side on shelves in alphabetical order, with alphabetical guides.
2 *Vertical* filing in multi-drawer cabinets which should have alphabetical guides on the outside of the drawers.
3 *Carousel* or rotary filing cabinets.

A tracer or marker card should always be inserted whenever a file is pulled, and removed once the medical record is back in place. The receptionist or secretary should always check to see whether a new continuation sheet is required for doctors to record their findings.

Whatever system of filing is used in the practice, accurate filing is essential. It should be possible to pull and refile records quickly and accurately.

Confidentiality of medical records

The medical record itself has a statement at the bottom saying it is the property of the Department of Health. However, the protection of the contents for purposes of confidentiality is the responsibility of the doctor and practice staff. Secretaries and receptionists must adhere to the rules of the practice established by the doctor as to who may access the information contained in the records.

Practice staff must never divulge any information contained in medical records and great care must be taken to ensure their safe custody. Remember, many people call into the practice and may be able to see over the reception counter and read things upside down. Cleaners and maintenance people may come into the practice when letters and other confidential information are left lying around.

There are certain legal issues appertaining to access to medical records, and data protection; these are explained fully in Chapter 4.

Much information about patients, their medical history, investigations, prescribing records, etc., are now stored on computer, but the principles of confidentiality still apply.

The medical record and information systems in general practice

The medical record is an important part of the overall information system for general practice. The record serves the needs of:

- preventive medicine
- at-risk groups of patients
- quality control measures – patient recall, performance review
- practice planning – administration and finance
- education – doctor, staff, trainee and patients
- research.

The age–sex register

The practice population can be well served by an age–sex register, either a manual system or computerized, to help identify patients at risk.

An age–sex register can be used for:

- child health surveillance
- child immunization uptake
- cervical cytology uptake
- geriatric screening (over 75s)
- hypertensive, diabetic, asthmatic patient screening (at-risk and chronic disease groups)
- health promotion
- an age–sex profile of the practice.

Disease or diagnostic index

Once again, the system of identification of patients who have certain diseases may be either maintained manually or stored as computer data. In its simplest form in a manual system, the notes can be colour-tagged according to the system established by the Royal College of General Practitioners, who have identified eight disease groups, for example:

- Red – sensitivities

- Brown – diabetes

- Yellow – epilepsy

- Green – tuberculosis

- Blue – hypertension

- White – long-term maintenance therapy

- Black – attempted suicide

- Black and white chequered – measles.

The presence of a coloured tag means that the disorder is, or has been, present; the absence of a tag can never imply the absence of such a disorder.

The medical records of deceased patients can either be sent back immediately to the health authority, or await their request for return of medical records on Form FP22. However, this procedure may change in the near future when medical practices are directly linked to health authorities by computer, when such procedures will be carried out by computer.

Report writing

Medical secretaries may be asked to investigate a procedure or system that is not running smoothly, or to give an account of an event or incident which has occurred.

Reports are written on a given subject to :

- convey information and ideas

- sometimes to convey recommendations.

The features of a good report are that:

- it is easily understood

- it is always clear

- it is as long as it needs to be, but no longer.

A report must be complete and accurate with regard to the information it conveys, and because a decision may be based on the report, it must be correct.

A logical structure of the type of report you may be asked to present would be:

- introduction

  – subject heading or title

  – terms of reference – what you have been asked to find out

  – procedure – how you found out

- body of report

  – findings – what you have found out

- conclusion

  – conclusions – your conclusion or diagnosis

  – recommendations – what you think should be done.

Medical secretaries may be asked to type more detailed reports, some of which may require a formal business format. There will, no doubt, be a 'house-style' which should be used, or reference to a manual of basic secretarial skills will give the necessary guidelines.

Note: A report must be accurate, clear, concise and logically arranged. It should be concise to the extent that there is no 'padding' or irrelevant details.

7

The hospital service

The patient's route through the hospital

The process begins with a visit, by the patient, either to their GP, or to an accident and emergency department (A&E), or to one of the few direct access services offered by some hospitals, for example walk-in clinics for genitourinary medicine. A GP visit results in a referral, leading to an outpatient appointment, a place on a waiting list and then admission. A direct visit to the hospital may result in a waiting list place or even immediate admission, with the GP being informed afterwards. Once in the hospital, the patient may be treated as an inpatient or a day case, with access as necessary to diagnostic services, operating theatres or treatment departments.

On discharge a summary of treatment given and follow-up needed is given to the patient's GP. Community support may be arranged, and follow-up clinic appointments may take place, either in the GP's surgery or back at the hospital itself, before the patient is fully discharged (Figure 7.1)

Outpatient appointments

A referral letter or specially designed referral form is sent by the GP to the appropriate consultant with an outline of the patient's condition. In exceptional circumstances, a telephone referral can be made. The consultant decides how urgent the case is, and when the patient should be seen. A letter or form is sent to the patient with details of the appointment.

If a patient has failed to turn up for a hospital appointment this is drawn to the attention of the consultant who decides whether another appointment is to be sent or whether the GP is to be informed first.

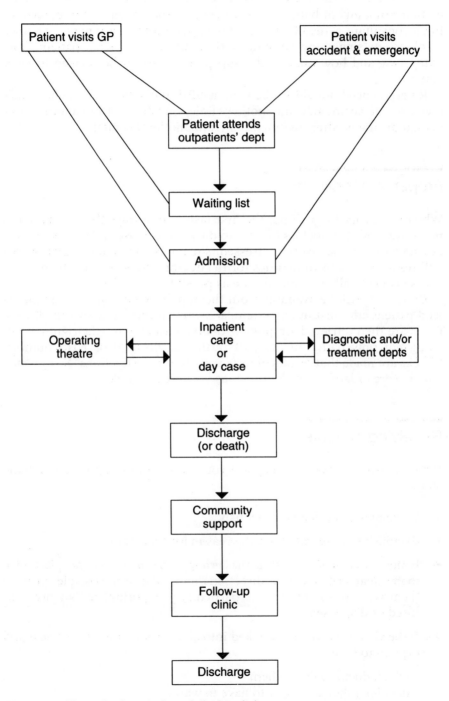

Figure 7.1   The patient's route through the hospital.

Outpatient appointments may be made centrally, or in each department, or in a mix of both. In many hospitals the system is computerized. Each consultant generally decides how appointments are made, whether in blocks or singly, the amount of time allocated to each patient, how many new and how many follow-up patients are to be booked in each clinic.

Referrals need not always be from a GP, but can be from the hospital's own A&E department, from another clinic, transferred from another consultant during or after treatment, or from another hospital.

Preparing for clinics

When preparing for a clinic, the first task is to ensure that the patient's notes are ready for doctors to refer to during the consultation. The importance of this cannot be over-stressed, since missing or incomplete notes will result in serious difficulties for the doctor and delays for the patient. It is sensible to allow as much time as possible.

Clinic lists will be available from the appointment book, or computerized patient administration system, showing all those due to attend. Case notes are then retrieved, or 'pulled', double-checking for the right patient using not only name but date of birth and hospital or NHS number. Checks are made that results of tests and other investigations, X-rays, etc., which were ordered after the previous visit are available.

Receiving patients

When a visitor arrives at reception you should go through the following stages:

- Smile and greet them courteously.

- Establish their identity and the reason for their visit.

- If the visitor has arrived at the wrong clinic in a busy hospital, give them clear and accurate directions and, wherever possible, provide them with an escort. This is particularly important if they are confused or distressed.

- If the visitor is a patient booked into clinic ask them to take a seat and explain to them:

  – which doctor will see them
  – how long they are likely to have to wait
  – where they can obtain refreshments
  – where the toilet is situated.

- Deal patiently and cheerfully with any queries the patient might have, and if you can't answer their questions yourself find someone (e.g. a nurse) who can.

- If there is likely to be any delay in the patient being seen, try to find out how long this is expected to be and give the patient a diplomatic and apologetic explanation.

- If the patient has language difficulties, obtain an interpreter or linkworker.

You should always be aware that the visitor may be experiencing discomfort or may be worried about the visit. This should be taken into account in all dealings with patients, their relatives and friends.

Admissions from the waiting list

Admissions from the waiting list (elective admissions) are usually handled by an admissions office, which is also responsible for keeping an accurate bed state for the entire hospital. Beds are not occupied at all times, although the hospital will try to maintain occupancy to the maximum to make best use of resources. Elective admissions will fill a portion of beds, but there must be the space and flexibility to be able to accommodate unforeseen demands. A pattern will have emerged over time, and the hospital will plan the use of its beds accordingly.

Admissions on to wards for day case treatment, to day surgery, or for the delivery of babies may be booked direct by those departments. Lists of expected admissions are given to each ward daily, and copied to the records department so that case notes are made available.

Accident and emergency admissions

When a patient is brought in to A&E by ambulance, the drivers will pass on whatever information they have obtained, and the receptionist will check what previous records exist for that patient. Treatment will not be delayed for this information if it is urgently needed. Particular procedures are followed if the patient is a road traffic accident victim, where ambulance transport costs are recovered, usually from the driver's insurance. Special arrangements also exist for suspected non-accidental injury of a child.

Every hospital has its own procedure for major accidents, and will rehearse it in conjunction with the emergency services, from time to time.

Follow-up after admission

When a patient is discharged from hospital the medical staff prepare a form for the patient to hand to their GP. A form is also completed for financial purposes, showing the diagnosis and any operations performed. After discharge a full summary is sent to the GP.

Not all patients leave the hospital alive. Following the death of a patient in general practice, the relatives must, of course, be dealt with in a kind and sensitive manner.

Day cases and ward attendees

More and more people opt for surgery as a day case, where this is possible. Strict criteria apply and not all procedures, or all patients can be dealt with in this way. Every effort is made to ensure that the patient has someone to collect them at the end of the day. An overnight stay will always be available should the patient's condition require it.

Most hospitals have taken steps to increase the proportion of work done on a day case basis, but interestingly, the assumption frequently made by patients that this is a cheaper option for the NHS is not often borne out. Many hospitals find that variable costs, for tests, disposables, etc. are higher per patient, and since they will be putting more patients through each bed, one per day rather than, for example, one per two or three days, total costs for these items can escalate. Staff costs can be higher because of the greater dependency of each patient, and the fixed costs associated with the building are not reduced until there has been a major shift from inpatients to day cases, allowing ward closures and large staff reductions.

The hospital team

Hospital staff fall into a number of professional groups, as follows:

Medical staff

- *Consultants* are responsible for the diagnosis and treatment of patients referred to them.

- *Junior doctors in training*, house officers, senior house officers, registrars and senior registrars, work for a consultant's firm. Although they are qualified doctors, they are in training for specialist roles.

- *Other doctors*, such as staff grades, clinical assistants, hospital practitioners and associate specialists are also attached to a consultant's firm. They are below consultant grade but are no longer in training.

Nursing staff

- *Nurses and midwives* carry out the regular care for patients as set out in the care plan, and administer drugs and treatment under the direction of the doctor. Psychiatric nurses work to ensure patients' mental health. Midwives care for mothers and babies and have special status as independent practitioners, which allows them in certain circumstances to practise without a doctor's prior instruction.

- *Health care assistants* and nursing assistants work with qualified nurses and therapists to deliver non-technical care to patients.

Therapy staff

- *Physiotherapists* diagnose and treat patients' difficulties with movement and rehabilitation after illness or injury, using exercises, manipulation and a range of equipment.

- *Occupational therapists* help patients to resume a normal life through activity based treatments, and the provision of aids to living, such as special tools and appliances.

- *Dieticians* advise patients and other care staff on the best food and drink for particular conditions. They also advise on intravenous and other drip feeding procedures.

- *Speech and language therapists* help patients with communication difficulties, especially after a stroke or other injury to the head, throat or chest. They also treat children who have communication difficulties.

- *Hearing therapists* assist patients with hearing difficulties and support those with hearing aids.

- *Pharmacists* provide specialist advice on appropriate drug treatments, including drug interactions, and supply drugs to inpatients and outpatients.

Diagnostic staff

- *Pathology* staff carry out a range of tests which are grouped into categories. Haematology staff carry out tests on blood, cytology staff study the nature of cells, especially cancerous or other diseased ones. Histology staff study tissues to detect disease. Microbiology staff test urine, faeces and other body fluids for parasites and bacteria, virology staff look for the presence of viruses, and chemistry staff look for the presence of chemicals which may cause illness or be a symptom of disease.

- *Radiography* staff take X-rays, for interpretation by a radiologist. They carry out various treatments, such as barium meals or dye injections, to show up particular parts of the body. They also use ultrasound to examine babies in the womb, and to detect disease, such as a tumour, in other parts of the body. Computerized axial tomography (CAT) scanning uses a computer to reconstruct an image of a layer of tissue in the body. Nuclear magnetic resource imaging (NMRI) uses radio frequency radiation and a magnetic field to produce anatomical sections of the body.

- *ECG* staff use an electrocardiograph to take readings which describe the functioning of a patient's heart, for cardiologists to interpret.

- *EEG* staff use an electroencephalograph to produce a picture of brain activity, placing small electrodes on the patient's head to measure electrical impulses. Consultants in EEG interpret the pictures.

Support workers

- *Non-clinical support departments* include chaplaincy, catering, cleaning, porters, security, building, engineering, linen and laundry, and transport.

Management and administration

- *Management departments* include the chief executive's team, general managers, directors of nursing and midwifery, business managers, personnel, finance, payroll, information and marketing.

- *Administrative support* is provided by admissions, registry and medical records.

Clinical audit

The term clinical audit embraces the audit activity of all health care professionals, including nurses, doctors and other health care staff. It is a widely used tool within hospitals, and is defined as the systematic and critical analysis of the quality of clinical care, including the procedures used for diagnosis, treatment and care, the associated resources and the resulting outcome and quality of life for the patient.

As a general principle, audit should be professionally led, and should focus on improving outcomes. It will have greatest impact if it forms part of routine clinical care. It should be seen as an educational process, and be an important part of quality programmes. It must respect confidentiality at the individual patient or clinician level and take into consideration the views of the patient and their carers.

What is a medical record?

A medical record is the history of a patient's treatment as an outpatient or inpatient, or both, at a particular hospital. If it is known that a patient has attended another hospital, a copy of that treatment record should be included in the current hospital medical record. A complete record prevents duplication and facilitates future care. In most cases, at present, the most complete medical records are the GP's notes as they follow patients as they move around. GP records should also contain details of any hospital treatment received by the patient, as well as any letters and summaries from hospitals which the patient may have attended.

Why have medical records in hospitals?

- The medical record is of most value in the treatment of patients, as a reminder and as a means of communication to doctors, nurses, etc., of what has been given and with what effect; and investigations which have been made and the results.

- They are an educational instrument and as such are used to teach medical students, nurses and other students.

- They are used for research.

Storage of medical records

Every hospital has its own system, but there are three main methods:

- lateral filing systems – files are side by side on shelves
- vertical filing systems – files are stored in multidrawer cabinets
- rotary (carousel) systems.

Each of these methods has advantages and disadvantages. Security of any area in which medical records are held is of prime importance.

Case notes

Although medical records were standardized when the NHS was instituted in order to ensure uniformity of record-keeping procedures, these vary from hospital to hospital. A hospital receptionist or medical secretary who moves from one hospital to another is unlikely to find herself handling exactly the same procedures. Standardization overall does exist but without rigidity.

Case notes basically follow the same pattern everywhere, being contained in A4-sized folders and consisting of five sections:

- identification
- medical
- nursing
- correspondence
- results, e.g. pathology tests, X-rays.

Identification section

This section allows space for the following information:

- hospital's name and code number, which is usually printed
- patient's name, address, status, telephone number
- patient's postcode
- date of birth
- GP information
- consultant
- hospital number
- occupation
- religion
- NHS number
- next of kin information.

Medical section

This section is for doctors' use only, and generally consists of:

- history of present complaint
- past medical history (PMH)
- family history
- patient complains of (PCO)
- on examination (OE)
- differential diagnosis
- investigations
- treatment.

Nursing section

This section contains the observations of nursing staff (recorded only when patients are admitted):

- nursing record

- temperature, pulse, respiration (TPR) – graphic records on special sheets. Also used for blood pressure, micturition and bowel function

- intake and output charts (record of all fluids taken orally or by transfusion and excreted).

Correspondence section

This section will usually include:

- GP's referral letter or proforma referral

- consultant's reports to GP

- letters to and from other consultants or other professionals.

Other information

The records may also contain:

- prescription charge

- social history

- theatre/surgical operation sheet

- consent form

- anaesthetic form.

The order of all these sheets inside the folder will vary from hospital to hospital, and ideally the order is printed either on the front or inside the cover. Each section of the case notes is generally filed in chronological order.

Master index

In theory, each patient should have only one medical record. This rule is broken by the law which states that the records of patients who attend the genitourinary clinics must be kept apart from any other medical records belonging to such patients. Also, psychiatric medical records of patients are usually kept separately with just a note placed in the main medical record stating where and when the patient attended for psychiatric care. In order to reduce the number of patients with several medical records, a master index is kept.

The master index is an alphabetical list of patients who have attended the hospital. It can be kept on cards and filed manually, on microfiche, on computer, on microfilm or on optic disc. The information recorded is usually basic: surname, forename(s), sex, date of birth, home address, marital status, sometimes date of first attendance and consultants seen, religion, date of death, patient index number.

The master index record for the accident and emergency and the emergency eye departments usually consists of alphabetically filed cards of attendees there.

Filing room/medical records library

This is the hub of the medical records department. It is often in a lower ground or ground floor because of the weight of all the records. Security in this area is of prime importance: unauthorized access cannot be allowed.

Within the library, files will be organized within a strict system. A number of different filing systems exist as follows, although in most hospitals medical records are filed by patient master index number. Colour coding is often used to prevent misfiling.

Master index number – terminal digit (12 34 **56**)

Six numbers are required. 12 34 **56** gives 56 as the terminal digit, 34 as the middle digit and 12 as the first digit. Divide the main area into 100 sections, 00 to 99, and these divisions give the foundation for terminal digit filing. This means that 56 will be in main section 56. The main sections are again divided into another 00 to 99 subsections, so 56 will be placed in subsection 34 and 12 will be placed behind 11 and before 13 in subsection 34. Though this may sound complicated, with a little practice it is easy to work and helps to cut down misfiling.

Middle digit (12 **34** 56)

A similar process to terminal digit is followed, but the numbers are followed in a different order.

- Straight numeric (1,2,3, etc.)

- Date of birth – alphabetic
- Surname – alphabetic.

Medical records procedures for departments

Accident and emergency records

If a patient arrives in hospital by emergency ambulance, the drivers will fill in the ambulance book giving what information about the patient they have collected. A receptionist will check if there are previous accident and emergency records and/or medical records, and will obtain them as quickly as possible. Treatment does not wait until these are found. If there is no record of previous attendance an A & E record is started with what information is available. This may be difficult if the patient is unconscious and unaccompanied, so there must be a follow-up should the patient eventually go onto a ward. Nurses usually record any property the patient is carrying, but a receptionist could be asked to do so, with a witness.

If the medical record shows that the patient has current appointments for outpatients, or has been booked for admission, or for theatre, these departments must be informed if the patient is not going to attend.

Outpatients records

Outpatients attend the hospital after a letter of referral from their GP. Many GPs use a referral form. This gives basic details of the patient which help to find any existing medical records. The letters go to the consultant or senior registrar of the department concerned and an appointment is given according to urgency. A list for each clinic is drawn up, and the medical records for all patients booked are then prepared.

A copy of the manual list or the computer list in 'pulling' order is produced. 'Pulling' is jargon for the actual gathering together of medical records from the filing shelves. Filing room staff, clinic clerks, receptionists or admission office staff may do this; again, this depends on each hospital's system.

The person preparing for the clinic will receive a copy of the list, and must obtain the medical records and laboratory tests, X-rays, etc. which were ordered at the previous visit. These results must be in the medical records and the X-rays ordered so that they are at the clinic. The medical records are also checked to ensure that there is paper on which the medical staff may write, and are 'stamped' or written up with the date and consultant of the clinic.

When the patient is new to the hospital the case notes are partially written up (in order to save paper and time) but details are not confirmed on the computer until the patient has actually arrived. On arrival all the patient details are checked and any missing information is obtained. Where a manual system is used this information is put on the master index card.

Day case records

These are usually handled by the department or the ward concerned. The medical records department is contacted for the necessary records before the patient arrives, where possible. The procedure is broadly the same as that described above for outpatients.

Maternity records

In many hospitals these records are retained by the woman throughout her pregnancy and only kept by the hospital after confinement.

Admissions and transfers

Lists of expected admissions are sent to each ward daily. A copy of this list is sent to the records library so that the medical records can be on the wards before the patient is admitted. Usually the ward receptionist does the check on the contents of the medical records, as described above for outpatients.

Retention of records

paediatric	25 years
mothers/babies	25 years
psychiatric	25 years
all others	8 years

The role of the secretary in hospital

The vital link

The secretary's role is a vital one in the smooth running of the department. Frequently the first point of contact, the secretary acts as representative of those for whom she works, and also represents the whole organization. She provides a link between members of the health care team, and between them and the outside world, and her involvement can ensure that scarce resources, such as a consultant's time or a theatre list, are used as efficiently as possible, and to the very best advantage. Diplomat, oiler of wheels, the one who gets things done, the one who remembers that important detail that everyone else has forgotten, the role is as varied as it is complex.

Core knowledge and skills

All secretarial posts in health care services require a body of core knowledge and skills which underpin all activities within the job. These include good interpersonal skills, respect for confidentiality, the ability to use appropriate medical terms, an understanding of the principles of medical ethics and etiquette, and sensitivity to the physical and psychological needs of patients and their carers.

In addition to these, there is a requirement to comply with legal requirements concerning working practices, and to be aware of and work within other health and safety regulations.

Key result areas

The role of each individual will vary, and the emphasis given to different parts of each job will be different, but the following key result areas are common to most:

COMMUNICATIONS	Processing, distribution and despatch of mail. Efficient and courteous use of communications systems, including telephone, answering machines, pagers, fax, telex and electronic mail.
CORRESPONDENCE	Identifying, prioritizing and responding to correspondence for own action, including letters, circulars, invoices and statements.

	Passing on correspondence for others' attention promptly.
ORGANIZING WORK SCHEDULES	Maintaining diaries, visual planners, computerized and other scheduling aids. Making and confirming appointments. Planning and prioritizing own work schedule. Co-ordinating assistance where necessary.
INFORMATION	Using manual and computerized filing systems. Responding to requests for and producing information from internal and external sources, including public documents, timetables, and statistics. Presenting information in different formats.
OFFICE ADMINISTRATION	Managing and controlling office stock, following appropriate ordering procedures. Dealing with faulty equipment. Maintaining a petty cash system.
MEETINGS	Preparing and producing agenda papers and minutes. Booking rooms, refreshments, and audio-visual aids. Arranging room layout. Attending meetings to take notes, and producing formal records of business undertaken.
RECEPTION	Receiving and screening visitors, and assisting them wherever possible.
DOCUMENTS AND REPORTS	Preparing and producing documents, including reports, tables and statistics. Arranging copying, collating and binding.
APPOINTMENT SYSTEMS	Answering requests for and allocating appointments. Following booking-in procedures, registration procedures, preparing case notes, paperwork, tests, results, etc. for clinics or surgical lists.
WAITING LISTS	Accurately compiling and prioritizing of waiting lists, manual or computerized. Arranging and confirming appointments, handling queries, and undertaking follow-up action as necessary.
HEALTH AND SAFETY	Ensuring the work area is kept free from hazards. Recording and reporting accidents and unsafe features. Following safe methods for lifting and handling

	heavy or bulky items. Following procedures for procedures for raising the alarm or summoning assistance. Adhering to procedures for handling specimens.
PATIENT CARE AND SUPPORT	Dealing with patients and carers with sensitivity, identifying and responding to their needs. Adhering to the requirements of the Patient's Charter. Arranging transport and escorts, following procedures for handling patients' property.

Private medicine

Introduction

A number of medical secretaries and receptionists are now employed in private medicine, either working for specialist physicians or surgeons in their consulting rooms, or in a private clinic or hospital.

Although, essentially, their function is similar to secretaries and receptionists working in NHS organizations, there are certain differences in working practice (see Chapters 6 and 7).

Private clinic or hospital

Patient contact and communication

Receptionists welcome patients on arrival at the clinic or hospital, where they may be asked to complete registration forms. They will take telephone calls from patients and advise them of payment protocol, make appointments for them to see a doctor, and if necessary refer to a nurse for advice.

Customer care

Customer care is always an important element in a private clinic. For example, tea or coffee is offered free of charge to patients waiting in outpatients.

In an effort to improve the quality of care, receptionists will present questionnaires to patients, who are asked to comment on all aspects of their care through the outpatient department including reception, nursing, X-ray, phlebotomy, etc.

Other aspects of customer care are the same as to be expected from a similar NHS organization, for example, arranging for a wheelchair or porter, and to generally help a patient as is felt necessary.

Telephone skills

In common with other areas of medical practice, the receptionist in a private clinic or hospital deals with all types of people – elderly, vague people, overseas visitors who cannot speak English very well, impatient people, demanding people. Patience, tact, understanding and a good telephone manner are just as essential in a private setting, as well as the ability to deal with situations efficiently and quickly because there is always another call waiting to be dealt with!

Appointments

When patients make appointments, they are asked for the basic information:

- name (surname and forename(s))
- age, if necessary
- telephone number
- address
- whether they have medical insurance.

An appointment card is sent to the patient with directions on how to reach the clinic, and details of car parking availability. The patient is informed of consultation costs (if known) and the cost of any investigations.

Outpatient hospital/clinic registration procedure

Patients are asked to complete a registration form on arrival at reception, giving the following information:

- name, address, telephone number
- name of consultant

- method of payment, and may be asked to sign that they are willing to pay for their treatment on the day.

Inpatient registration

If a patient has to be admitted, a more detailed form is given to them for completion, which also asks for details of their insurance cover.

In some private clinics, patients may be encouraged to pay for outpatient treatment on the day of their appointment, and to get any insurance forms signed there and then by the consultant, so that there will be little or no delay in reimbursement.

Pathology and X-ray

Receptionists may generate accounts for patients attending for pathology and X-ray, and will request payment at the time of investigation.

Medical records

Consultants in a private hospital or clinic will bring patients' notes with them, and keep them in their personal possession.

The only records kept at the clinic will be screening records such as well-woman, executive screening, breast screening, etc. All records of work generated by the staff are retained at the clinic.

Mail – incoming and outgoing

Mail addressed to doctors is generally kept in pigeon-holes for their collection. All outgoing mail, accounts, letters, etc. are collected by the mail room at the end of the day for posting.

Patient accounts

Preparation and processing of patient accounts is a major part of the receptionist's job. They are prepared on the computer, and have to be ready for patients when they leave the clinic. Private hospitals and clinics have the facility to collect cash, accept payment by credit cards and cheques, and often have a 'switch' machine.

Systems

All accounts for the day will be sent to a main accounts department for filing. Any outstanding bills can be demonstrated on the computer screen. There is a variety of software available, but a frequently used system is 'Compucare'.

Liaison with other health care professionals

Receptionists have regular contact with consultants and their secretaries, as well as with physiotherapy, X-ray and nursing staff at the clinic. They will have frequent telephone contact with almost every cross-section of the medical field, including laboratory staff, doctors, secretaries, NHS hospitals, clinics (private and NHS), psychologists, etc.

From time to time, they may be asked to contact a patient's private medical insurance company for information regarding levels of cover, etc.

Waiting areas and consulting rooms

Consulting rooms are checked and maintained by nursing staff, except for stationery items, which are the responsibility of the receptionists.

Doctors will usually liaise by telephone to ask for their patients to be taken to them, and the receptionist or nurse will show them into the doctors' rooms.

Waiting areas are kept clean and tidy by frequent visits from house-keepers. Catering staff will ensure a supply of tea and coffee and remove dirty cups from the waiting area. Magazines are always available for patients.

The secretary in private practice

The role of the secretary in private practice is a diverse and varied one, requiring qualities and skills additional to secretarial duties. In many instances, the secretary will be working on her own apart from the days her consultant is seeing patients at the practice. This means that decisions of a non-medical nature may have to be made.

Reception and secretarial duties

A great deal of the secretary's time is involved with answering the telephone, dealing with patients' enquiries and making appointments.

Once an appointment is made for a new patient, a file is made up with basic patient information and details of private medical insurance cover, in readiness for the initial consultation.

The secretary may be asked by her consultant to organize investigations (pathology, radiological, etc.) for patients when necessary and to arrange for external referrals, for example, physiotherapy, other consultants. Admission to hospital or clinic may also be arranged for the patient.

From time to time the secretary will need to liaise with her NHS counterpart, either to leave a message or to contact the consultant when he/she is working in the hospital department.

She will be responsible for keeping the consulting room, waiting room and her own office tidy and generally ensuring the comfort of patients while they wait to see the doctor.

Clerical duties

On a daily basis mail has to be sorted and incoming correspondence attended to as appropriate. Photocopying of insurance or medical reports may have to be done from time to time, and messages sent or received by facsimile (fax) transmission accordingly dealt with. Correspondence will have to be posted and a supply of postage stamps maintained at the practice.

The secretary will usually be responsible for petty cash to purchase office sundries and maintain supplies of stationery and other items.

Patients records will be pulled prior to consultation and checked that results of investigations previously requested are complete. Following consultation and any further action that has to be taken, the notes will be filed away.

Secretarial skills

Good secretarial skills are important, including typing and competent use of wordprocessing systems. Many consultants prefer to dictate their letters and reports onto a dictating machine, but some still prefer their secretaries to use shorthand. Usually, a combination of both shorthand and audiotyping is desirable.

A knowledge of medical terminology and medical abbreviations are always useful, but not necessarily essential. A good medical dictionary, commonsense and an ability to learn the specialist terms will usually suffice.

In private practice, with no nurse in attendance, the secretary may find that she is asked to act as a chaperone during the consultant's examination of the patient.

Practice Management

The secretary in private practice will find that in addition to her other duties she is also a practice manager. The good manager will update existing systems to ensure the practice operates effectively and in an efficient way. She will be responsible for sending patient accounts, and if necessary, will remind patients that settlement of their outstanding account is overdue, and will follow up unpaid accounts on a regular basis, as well as patient account reconciliation. Any long-standing overdue accounts will be referred to a debt collection agency when necessary.

The secretary will reconcile the petty cash account on a regular (usually monthly) basis, and recommend when accounts should be paid by the consultant.

Another financial aspect of the work of the medical secretary in private practice will, no doubt, be to operate a payroll (maybe for one person only), to calculate her own PAYE and NI contributions, and to make year end returns to the Inland Revenue. She will also be responsible for ordering any supplies necessary for the doctor's consulting room and her own office requirements.

Summary

It will be noted that the role of the receptionist and secretary in private practice is very much the same as working in an NHS organization.

An essential quality is to be able to deal with patients in an efficient yet sympathetic manner, and understand the emotions and concerns experienced by patients when entering a clinical environment. Although it is desirable for secretaries and receptionists to have a knowledge of medical terminology and other clinical aspects, a competent person will learn these as they carry out their day-to-day duties.

9

Forms, fees and finances in general practice

Introduction

General medical practice is a small business, like any other practice of professionals e.g. solicitors or accountants. Therefore there is a need to get money in to cover the costs of providing the service to patients. Figure 9.1 shows a list of expenses incurred in running a practice and a list of sources of income. The profit is the difference between income and expenditure, and it is from the profit that the partners take their drawings. It is therefore easy to understand why doctors insist that all claims for payments are made promptly and that expenses are kept down to a minimum.

The majority of the income is via the FHSA/health board, and in order to claim their share a practice has to complete a variety of forms – these are the equivalent of invoices for services given. Whilst some of the forms are filled in only when a partner joins a practice, or on an annual basis, the majority are completed as each service is rendered. Therefore, the receptionist is a key person in ensuring that forms are completed as patients enter or leave the premises. Figure 9.2 shows the items of income set against the staff members who may be responsible for ensuring the claim forms are completed.

Practices have a variety of ways of sharing out the clerical workload, and in larger practices it may be expedient to have one or two staff who take responsibility for checking that forms are completed and sent off to the FHSA/health board on a weekly basis. However, if all the receptionists are good at completing the forms accurately and completely the task of batching and sending off becomes much easier and quicker.

Most practices have systems for ensuring that forms are filled in at the right time, these will range from stickers on the outside of the medical record, through cardex boxes (manual recording) to computer generated

Income

NHS	Practice Allowance	
	Capitation	Registration
		Child health surveillance
		Deprivation
	Items of service	Registration medical
		Night visits
		Maternity services
		Emergency treatment
		Immediately necessary treatment
		Contraceptive services
		Temporary residents
		Adult vaccination/immunization
		Minor surgery
	Targets	Cervical cytology
		Immunizations under 2s
		Immunizations under 5s
	Health promotion banding	
	Dispensing payments	
	Associate allowance	
	Seniority	
	Postgraduate education allowance	
	Trainee supervision grant	
	Medical students	
	Reimbursements	Trainee salary
		Rent and rates
		Staff salaries and NI
		Staff training
		Computer maintenance
Private	Private medical attendant reports	
	Insurance medicals	
	Cremation forms	
	Sundry	Passport forms
		Travel vaccinations, e.g. yellow fever
		PSV, HGV, elderly driver
	Other appointments	Company or school medical officer
		Police surgeon

Expenditure

Practice	Drugs and instruments
	Hire and maintenance of equipment
	Repairs and renewals
Premises	Rates and water rates
	Heat and light
	Insurance
	Cleaning
Salaries	Staff
	Trainee
Administration	Postage
	Stationery
	Telephone
Professional fees	Accountant
	Solicitor
Banking	Interest
	Loan repayments

The turnover (i.e. all forms of income added together) of a large practice may be in excess of £500 000 whereas that of a small single-handed practice might be £90 000.
These figures exclude budgets for fundholding and any monies received by practices to manage fundholding.

Figure 9.1 Practice income and expenditure.

Source of income	Item	Persons likely to complete the claim form			
		Receptionist	Clerk	Secretary	Manager
NHS	Practice allowance	automatic (only affected by change of partnership)			
	Capitation				
	Registration	✔	✔		
	Child health surveillance	✔	✔		
	Deprivation	automatic (depends upon post code)			
	Items of service				
	Registration medical	✔			
	Night visits	✔	✔		
	Maternity services	✔			
	Emergency treatment	✔			
	Immediately necessary treatment	✔			
	Contraceptive services	✔			
	Temporary residents	✔			
	Adult vaccination/ immunization	✔			
	Minor surgery	✔	✔		
	Targets				
	Cervical cytology	✔	✔		
	Immunizations under 2s	✔	✔		
	Immunizations under 5s	✔	✔		
	Health promotion banding		✔		✔
	Dispensing payments		✔		
	Associate allowance			✔	✔
	Seniority	automatic once set up			✔
	Postgraduate education allowance			✔	✔
	Trainee supervision grant			✔	✔
	Medical students			✔	✔
	Reimbursements				
	Trainee salary				✔
	Rent and rates			✔	✔
	Staff salaries and NI				✔
	Staff training				✔
	Computer maintenance				✔
Private	Private medical attendant reports			✔	✔
	Insurance medicals			✔	
	Cremation forms			✔	
	Sundry				
	Passport forms	✔			
	Travel vaccinations, e.g. yellow fever	✔			
	PSV, HVG, elderly driver	✔			
	Other appointments				
	Company or school medical officer			✔	
	Police surgeon			✔	

Figure 9.2   Income in general practice and the role of the receptionist.

lists and reminder messages on the computer screen when a patient record is opened. The introduction of FHSA/GP links project where claims can be sent automatically to the FHSA/health board will eventually make the paper claims redundant.

Regardless of the system of claiming it is important that receptionists are aware of what claims should be made under what circumstances. Various publications exist to give information on capitation, item of service claims, targets and payments to doctors. The most important is the Red Book – the Statement of Fees and Allowances. This is a loose-leaf document, which is updated as rates of pay, conditions regulating payments, or other changes are made, and the FHSA/health board base their decisions regarding payments on its content. Every partner and trainee GP in a practice is issued with their own copy of the Red Book, and every surgery needs to have a copy available to receptionists who want to check what is payable and when. Furthermore, it is essential that all copies of the Red Book are kept up to date, so that when the latest statement of fees and allowances (SFA) (amendment to the Red Book) is issued the new pages are appropriately filed into place and the old versions disposed of.

To understand what can be claimed under which circumstances there is no real substitute for reading the Red Book and clarifying queries with the FHSA/health board. Many FHSAs run short courses so that surgery staff can learn what the forms are for, how they should be completed, when to return them to the FHSA/health board, and so on. Alternatively, it is possible to make an appointment to go to the FHSA/health board to meet the staff who deal with claims. The receptionist who has made friends with people in the FHSA/health board with whom regular contact has to be made is most likely to be able to submit claims accurately, promptly and keep abreast of trends and changes. There are so many changes affecting both surgeries and FHSAs/health boards these days that 'networking' is an essential activity.

In the surgery a collection of claim forms can be put into a folder along with brief details of when claims should be made, notes on completing the forms, and in-house systems for recording 'due to sign again' dates. This is a useful in-house reference source and training tool for new staff. However, as and when changes are made to claims it is important to ensure that the folder is updated.

It is important when handling claim forms and target sheets to be systematic, and therefore it is preferable not to work on reception duties at the same time, trying to squeeze in the paperwork between other tasks. Paperwork takes a different set of skills to those used in receiving patients. If a receptionist works a busy morning shift on the reception desk it will be almost impossible to switch from pressured reception duties to calmly working through a pile of papers without a transitory period – cup of coffee, pop out to the shops for fresh air, a chat, to wind down from the pressure.

RECEPTION DESK DUTIES	CLERICAL DUTIES
Require the ability to juggle many important priorities all at one time	Require a systematic orderly approach
Answering the telephone, controlling surgery flow and dealing with queries are 'demand driven' activities	Processing massive piles of paper requires self motivation – 'self driven'

Practice income

Income to the practice is derived from NHS sources, and from private sources, e.g. item of service claim forms come via the NHS, medical attendant reports for insurance companies are a private source (see Figure 9.1).

The fees payable for NHS payments are shown in the Red Book and the BMA recommend fees for private services. Both these sets of fees are summarized and displayed in tabular form in the doctor's weekly or monthly magazines.

It is important that all sources of income are properly documented and claimed. The role of the receptionist cannot be underestimated in ensuring that services given are recorded and claimed for. The receptionist is the person who deals with the patients, is aware of what the doctor says he/she has done for a specific patient, and therefore is the pivotal person to ensure that claims are made or invoices are raised. The receptionist may not be required to do these tasks but to ensure that someone else has the necessary information to be able to do so.

However, there will be occasions when a receptionist is asked to advise a patient of what payment is required, to receive the payment and issue a receipt. Information about current fees should be kept readily to hand, along with printed receipts that need only to have name of patient, service given, date, amount paid and signature filled in by hand. The payment should then be passed to the appropriate person for banking.

Although most doctors are aware that private fees are a significant supplement to their income, some are reluctant to talk to patients about the fee for their services. Also staff should be aware that sums received from patients, great and small, cheque or cash, must all be passed through the practice accounts. Private fees are not a 'perk' – the Inland Revenue have been known to trace payments back over a number of years and claim back tax on them.

As in all the other aspects of general medical practice, the receptionist has a vital role to play in the financial success of a practice by cutting down on unnecessary wastage and expense, and ensuring that all income is claimed and processed promptly.

Helpful hints in completing FHSA claim forms

The following information should help you in completing any claim forms for which you are responsible in your practice.

Application to go on a doctor's list (FP54, FP4, FP1)

When a baby is born a parent has to register the birth. They go to the Registrar of Births, Deaths and Marriages with the birth certificate. A small pink card (FP54) is issued to the parent. This card has the registration of birth number on it and this will, until death, be the National Health number of that person.

To register the new baby with a GP the parent takes the pink FP54 card to a doctor and asks to join the list. If the doctor accepts he signs the pink card and sends it to his administration – the FHSA or health board. They in turn send a medical card (FP4) to the parent which contains all the baby's details together with the name of the GP. At the same time the FHSA send the GP a new FP6/7 (Medical Record envelope) which shows the patient's name, date of birth, address, National Health Service number together with the date the baby was registered with the GP. Everyone living in Great Britain is entitled to an individually numbered medical card. It is retained by the person and whenever they change GPs they sign it and hand it in to the new GP. The new GP in turn signs the medical card of his newly accepted patient and sends it off to his FHSA/health board, who in turn issue a new medical card with the existing NHS number but now showing the new GP's details . This is sent to the patient. However, if a medical card is lost or destroyed, to join a GP's list an 'Application to join a Doctor's list' form has to be completed (Figure 9.3).

For every registration a fee is paid to a GP by the FHSA/health board. Not only that, once it is received by the FHSA/health board it enables them to trace the previous GP and request him to forward all medical records, they in turn send the notes to the new GP thus enabling a person's medical notes to stay with them from birth to death irrespective of how many GPs they have registered with during their lives.

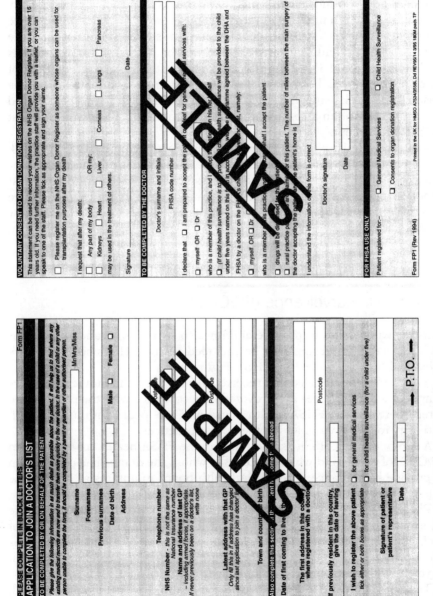

Figure 9.3 Application to join a doctor's list – FPY1.

Registration fee claim (FP/RF)

When a patient who is five years old or older registers with a GP, the GP must offer in writing to carry out a health promotion consultation. If a patient is housebound the GP must offer to travel to their home to carry this out. If there is a practice nurse she can carry out the assessment. A fee will then be paid to the GP if the consultation is carried out within three months of the patient registering. A fee *may* be paid if the assessment is carried out between 3 – 12 months after registration if through no fault of his own, the GP has been unable to carry out an assessment earlier. The reason for the delay must be entered on the FP/RF form. It has been found that if the offer of an assessment is made at the time of registration most patients will accept.

As a receptionist you will be responsible for offering this health check assessment and are asked to bear in mind that a fee is paid to the GP for every assessment made. After each assessment the patient's details must be added to the claim form (there is room for 20 patient details) and once the form is complete it should be sent to the FHSA/health board and a new form started (Figure 9.4).

Child health surveillance (FP/CHS)

A doctor who wishes to provide child health surveillance and be paid for such services should apply to be included in the FHSA's/health board's child health surveillance list (CHS) (Figure 9.5).

A doctor on the CHS list will receive a fee for each child under five years of age for whom services are provided in accordance with the programme agreed between the FHSA/health board and the local community health authority for the area in which the doctor practices.

A doctor on the CHS list should inform the FHSA/health board, on form FP/CHS, of each child who registers for whom the doctor has undertaken to provide surveillance. The FHSA/health board maintains a list of these children separate from the normal general medical services patient list.

There is one level of fee, and this is paid automatically according to the information provided by the doctor on form FP/CHS on the first day of each quarter. Payment is made whether or not any particular service has been provided in respect of the child during the preceding quarter. Payment will cease once the child is five.

The service comprises: monitoring the health, well being and physical, mental and social development of the child while under the age of five years with a view to detecting any deviations from normal development.

The GP should keep an accurate record of the development of the child under the age of five years, compiled as soon as it is reasonably

FP/RF
(MULTI)
NHR01902

Registration fee claim

Fill in this form for patients aged 5 or over who you or your partner(s) have
* *accepted onto your/their list and*
* *for whom you/they have carried out all the examination procedures specified in paragraph 13B(2) of the Terms of Service.*

The examination should normally be carried out within 3 months of you or your partner(s) inviting the patient to participate in a consultation.

The FHSA may ask the patient, parents or guardian to confirm the information on this form.

For more information, see SFA 23.

Details of claiming GP

Surname

Initials

FHSA Code Number

Declaration

I declare

* that the information on this form is correct

* that I/my partner(s) have carried out all the examination procedures described in paragraph 13B(2) of the Terms of Service

* that I/my partner(s) am not claiming in respect of a patient who was immediately before joining my/their list, a patient of a partner, and who participated in an examination under paragraph 13B of the Terms of Service during the 12 months before joining my/their list.

I claim payment in accordance with the Statement of Fees and Allowances.

Doctor's Signature

Date

Practice Stamp

Figure 9.4   Registration fee claim form – FP/RF.

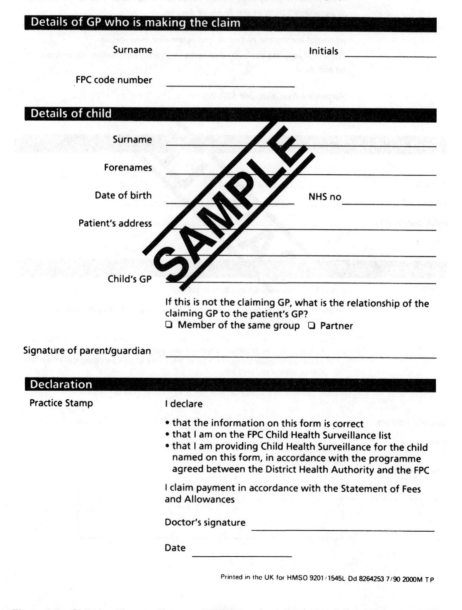

FP/CHS

Child health surveillance fee claim

Fill in one of these forms for each child for whom you have undertaken to provide Child Health Surveillance
For more information, see SFA paragraph 22

Details of GP who is making the claim

Surname _____ Initials _____

FPC code number _____

Details of child

Surname _____

Forenames _____

Date of birth _____ NHS no _____

Patient's address _____

Child's GP _____

If this is not the claiming GP, what is the relationship of the claiming GP to the patient's GP?
❑ Member of the same group ❑ Partner

Signature of parent/guardian _____

Declaration

Practice Stamp

I declare

• that the information on this form is correct
• that I am on the FPC Child Health Surveillance list
• that I am providing Child Health Surveillance for the child named on this form, in accordance with the programme agreed between the District Health Authority and the FPC

I claim payment in accordance with the Statement of Fees and Allowances

Doctor's signature _____

Date _____

Printed in the UK for HMSO 9201/1545L Dd 8264253 7/90 2000M T P

Figure 9.5   Child health surveillance – FP/CHS.

practicable following the first examination and provide the community health authority with a statement of procedures undertaken in the course of the examination.

Notification of child surveillance (SUR/01/90)

This form is to be used by GPs and community health staff to notify the FHSA/health board of child surveillance activity (Figure 9.6). It will be used to ensure that coverage is adequate.

The top copy is sent to the FHSA/health board who forward it on to the community trust. The second copy is retained by the GP for his/her own records, and the third copy may be used by the parent/guardian who may wish to keep their own record.

The following sections of the form need to be completed:

1   date of contact
2   all child's details
3   professional's details
4   tick appropriate surveillance stage, e.g. eight weeks
5   enter correct code in the boxes for the individual checks
6   tick any result or action taken
7   send completed form to FHSA/health board as soon as completed.

Adult vaccination claims (FP73 (MULTI))

This form provides for up to 20 adult vaccination claims at a time. It should not be used for patients aged 16 years or under. Please ensure the reason vaccination is given is entered on the form (Figure 9.7).

Vaccination claims (FP73)

This form should be used for vaccination claims for non-targeted children (i.e. 5 – 16 years) (Figure 9.8).

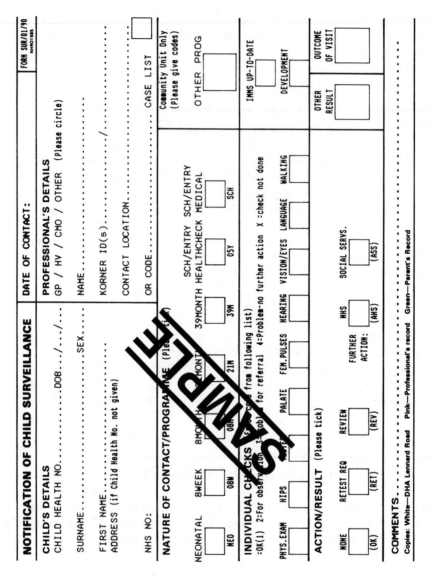

Figure 9.6 Notification of child surveillance – SUR/01/90.

ADULT VACCINATION AND IMMUNISATION CLAIM (not for childhood immunisations)

Surname & Initials	Address	NHS No.	Date of Birth	Antigen	Batch No.	1, 2, 3 Reinf	Date Given	Reason (see below)	FP19 Y/N	FHSA use
1.										
2.										
3.										
4.										
5.										
6.										
7.										
8.										
9.										

SAMPLE

PRACTICE STAMP

REASONS CODES: (a) routine measure (b) belonging to a group exposed to special risk (c) traveller abroad
(please enter name of country with code)
(d) recommended by the Community Physician/Proper Officer during an out break of disease.

CLAIMING DOCTOR .... SIGNATURE ....

Figure 9.7 Adult vaccination claims – FP73 (MULTI).

FP 73 (Revised 12/88)

VACCINATION AND IMMUNISATION ATTENDANCE AT: CLINIC/SURGERY:

SURNAME: SEX: MALE/FEMALE

FORENAMES: D.O.B.:

ADDRESS: POST CODE:

SCHOOL: NHS NO.:   CHILD HEALTH NO.: □ □ □ □ □ □

GENERAL PRACTITIONER'S SURNAME AND INITIALS:

HEALTH VISITOR'S CASE LIST NO.: □ □ □   (OR HV'S NAME:)

I consent to my child receiving   Poliomyelitis   Diphtheria   Tetanus   Whooping   Measles   Mumps   Rubella
the following immunisations: Cough

                                      □   □   □   □   □   □   □

Signature of Parent of Guardian .... Date ....

TO BE COMPLETED BY PERSON ADMINISTERING IMMUNISATION:

Primary Courses		BATCH NO.	DOSE	DATE	NAME	DESIG.	STAFF ID NO.
First Dose	Diphtheria						
	Tetanus						
	Pertussis						
	Poliomyelitis						
Others (please 1.							
specify) 2.							
Second Dose	Diphtheria						
	Tetanus						
	Pertussis						
	Poliomyelitis						
Others (please 1.							
specify) 2.							
Third Dose	Diphtheria						
	Tetanus						
	Pertussis						
	Poliomyelitis						
Others (specify)	Measles						
	Mumps						
	Rubella						
Boosters	Diphtheria						
	Tetanus						
	Polio						
Others (please 1.							
specify) 2.							

Date and Result of any test of Immunity for Rubella

Comments:

TO BE COMPLETED BY GENERAL PRACTITIONER CLAIMING PAYMENT

Vaccinated as □   (a) A routine Measure   Name and address of
                                                                     General Practitioner
               □   (b) Belonging to a group exposed to special risk   (BLOCK CAPITALS OR STAMP)

(Please tick) □   (c) A traveller to .... (Name of Country)

               □   (d) Recommended by the Proper Officer during an outbreak of disease

I certify that the patient has been vaccinated as indicated above and I claim the appropriate fees.

Date .... Signature of Doctor ....
                                                                     No: □ □ □ □ □

Signature of Assistant or Locum on behalf of Doctor ....

PLEASE SUBMIT THIS FORM TO THE IMMUNISATION DEPARTMENT, 12-18 LENNARD ROAD, AS SOON AS EACH DOSE IS
GIVEN. PLEASE DO NOT WAIT FOR COMPLETION OF A COURSE.

SAMPLE

Figure 9.8   Vaccination claims – FP73.

Notification of immunizations for targeted children (five years and under) (FP/73/3/GP and FP73/2/GP)

Form FP/73/3/GP (primary immunizations)

This form is in four parts. The top sheet records the child's personal details and the first dose of immunization and, once completed, should be sent to the FHSA – the remaining parts are retained to record the second and third doses. The second sheet retains the details from the first sheet and provides space for the second dose details. Once completed, this sheet should be sent to the FHSA. The third sheet retains details from the first two sheets and provides space for the third dose to be recorded and it should then be passed on as before. The remaining sheet (card) is the file copy and is for retention by the GP for inclusion in his/her files (Figure 9.9).

Form FP/73/2/GP (MMR, boosters and ad hoc)

This form is in two parts. Once completed the top sheet should be passed on to the FHSA – the remaining sheet is the file copy and can be used by the GP for his/her records (Figure 9.10).

Figure 9.9   Notification of immunizations for targeted children – FP/73/3/GP.

IMMUNISATION RECORD						
Surname		Forenames		Sex M/F	D O B	CHS No.
Address				Surgery/Clinic/Home		
GP Name & Initials		HV Name		HV (CHS) No.		NHS No.

NOT FOR PRIMARY IMMUNISATIONS

Measles ☐ Poliomyelitis ☐ Whooping Cough ☐
Mumps ☐ Diphtheria ☐ Hib ☐
Rubella ☐ Tetanus ☐ ☐

CONSENT ... WITH PARENTAL RESPONSIBILITY:
...sent to ... receiving these immunisations

Sig: .... Date: ....

DELETE ANTIGENS NOT GIVEN

ANTIGEN	BATCH No.	DATE	ME		STAFF ID OR DESIGNATION
Measles					
Mumps					
Rubella					
BOOSTERS					
Diphtheria					
Tetanus					
Polio					
OTHER					
Hib					

Date and Result of any test of immunity for Rubella:

FP/73/2/GP (Revised 2/92)

Figure 9.10   Notification of immunizations of targeted children – FP/73/2/GP.

Night visit claim form (FP/81)

All night visits must be entered onto form FP/81 – there is space for ten individual visits to be listed. Once the form is completed it is to be sent to the FHSA and a new form made available for further entries (Figure 9.11).

Some GPs prefer to carry these forms themselves and thus take the responsibility of entering any night visits they may do. If it is the receptionist's duty to ensure all sections of the form are completed, remember the following points:

- The patient need not sign the form.

- The patient must be registered – either fully registered, temporary resident, immediate necessary treatment or maternity care.

- A night fee can be claimed for calls requested and made between 10 pm and 8 am.

- A lower fee is paid if a GP working on behalf of a commercial deputizing service makes the night visit.

- If more than one patient is seen at the same address enter all their details as a fee is paid for all claims (first two paid at same rate, for the

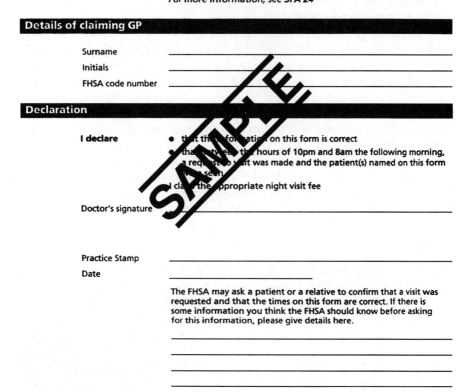

Figure 9.11   Night visit claim form – FP/81.

next three patients half the full rate is paid and any subsequent patients a fee of one tenth of full rate is paid).

Contraceptive services (FP1001, FP1002 and FP1003)

A GP can claim a fee for providing contraceptive services; an ordinary fee and a intrauterine device fee (coil). The FHSA pay an annual fee for services and every three months they pay the GP a quarter of the annual fee.

If a GP fits an intrauterine device, the first quarter's payment is at a higher rate than the other three quarterly payments. Any woman (not only a woman registered for general medical services) can apply to be accepted as a contraceptive patient.

The ordinary fee is paid (FP1001) when a GP accepts a patient, gives advice and conducts any necessary examination, prescribes drugs or a cap and provides any necessary follow-up care. Even if a woman attends the surgery and advice is given about a male contraceptive or vasectomy, a GP may still claim if he/she accepts responsibility for the after care of the female patient (Figure 9.12).

Intrauterine device: (FP1002) – A GP can claim the intrauterine device fee for services provided to a woman during the 12-month period beginning from the day she applies to have the device fitted. The fee is paid only if the GP or partner fits the device and gives all necessary after care including any replacement for the next 12 months. It is not possible to claim this fee in addition to the ordinary fee. Twelve months after insertion of the device, the ordinary fee will become payable for any period during which a device is not replaced (Figure 9.13).

Temporary resident patients: (FP1003) – If contraceptive service is required a GP can claim and he/she will be paid one quarter of the annual fee. If it is a temporary resident having an intrauterine device fitted he/she will be paid one half of the annual intrauterine device fee (Figure 9.14).

Remember

Claims should be made on form FP1001 for the ordinary contraceptive fee and on FP1002 if an intrauterine device has been fitted. Whichever form is applicable it has to be signed by the patient and the top copy retained by the patient as a reminder to sign again in 12 month's time.

Temporary resident claims are made on FP1003 and must be signed by the patient.

At the end of 12 months a new claim must be sent to the FHSA/health board for each patient for whom contraceptive services are continuing. If a patient comes to the surgery for contraceptive services within one month of the date on which the 12 month period will end, a new form can be completed and submitted to the FHSA which will accept it as taking effect from the end of the 12-month period. If a patient does not attend at about the time the 12-month period ends but does so within 18 months of the first claim a GP can still claim that the service has been continuous and the FHSA will pay retrospectively for the missing quarters. For instance, if a patient was first accepted in May 1990 but did not attend again until September 1991 seeking renewal of contraceptive services, the claim can be regarded as being submitted in May 1991. A GP will cease to be paid for a patient as soon as the FHSA receives a subsequent claim from another doctor.

The bottom section of the FP1001 may be kept in the patient's notes as a reminder to the GP as to when the 12-month period ends.

**NATIONAL HEALTH SERVICE
CONTRACEPTIVE SERVICES
PART I**
(to be detached and given to the patient)

Patient's name ....

You have been accepted for contraceptive services by Dr ....
for the 12 months ending on .... 199 ....

Please bring this slip with you the first time you visit the doctor for contraceptive services
after that date. If you change to another doctor for contraceptive services please take this
slip with you.   Form FP 1001

**NATIONAL HEALTH SERVICE
PART II
APPLICATION FOR CONTRACEPTIVE SERVICES**
(to be completed by the patient)

To Dr ....

NAME (surname first) AND ADDRESS	(Name in BLOCK LETTERS please)
Date of birth	NHS Number (if known)
Former name(s) (if applicable)	

I apply to be accepted for contraceptive services for 12 months

Have you received contraceptive services from another doctor in the last 12 months?
                                                                        YES/NO

If YES, please give the doctor's name and address
      Name: Dr ....
      Address: ....
                    ....

Signed: .... Date ....

*Delete whichever does not apply   Form FP 1001

PART III
(to be retained by the doctor)
CONTRACEPTIVE SERVICES

NAME (surname first) AND ADDRESS		
	Date accepted	
	Date claim sent to FHSA	
	Renewal date	

                                                                        Form FP 1001

Figure 9.12   Contraceptive services – FP1001.

PART IV

DOCTOR'S CERTIFICATE AND CLAIM FOR PAYMENT

To.. FAMILY HEALTH SERVICES AUTHORITY

I undertake to give contraceptive services to the person named overleaf for 12 months, having regard to and being guided by modern authoritative medical opinion such as the advice given in the Handbook of Contraceptive Practice issued by the Standing Medical Advisory Committee.

I claim the appropriate fee.

Tick box
if   [   ]   I previously accepted this patient for contraceptive services
appropriate   in .... (date)

               [   ]   The claim is made after the due date for renewal and I certify
                             that services have been given continuously since that date.
                             I apply for payment to be continuous.

	Name and address of doctor or partnership.	For use by FHSA
Signed		
Date		

SAMPLE

Printed in the UK for HMSO. 11/91. Dd.DH000318. C750. 29637.

Figure 9.12   *Continued*

NATIONAL HEALTH SERVICE   **CONTRACEPTIVE SERVICES**

PART I

(to be detached and given to the patient)

Patient's name ....

You have been accepted for contraceptive services by Dr. ....

for the 12 months ending on .... 199 ....

Please bring this slip with you the first time you visit the doctor for contraceptive services after that date. If you change to another doctor for contraceptive services please take this slip with you.

Form FP 1002

NATIONAL HEALTH SERVICE

PART II

FITTING OF INTRA-UTERINE DEVICE

(to be completed by the patient)

To Dr. ....

NAME (surname first) AND ADDRESS   (Name in BLOCK LETTERS please)
Date of birth   N.H.S. number (if known)
Former name(s) (if applicable)

I have been advised to be fitted with an intra-uterine device.

Have you received contraceptive services from another doctor in the last 12 months?   *YES/NO*

If YES, please give the doctor's name and address

Name: Dr. ....

Address: ....

....

Signed: ....   Date ....

*Delete whichever does not apply   Form FP 1002

PART III

(to be retained by the doctor)

FITTING OF INTRA-UTERINE DEVICE

NAME (surname first) AND ADDRESS		
	Date IUD fitted	
	Date claim sent to FPC	
	Renewal date	

Form FP 1002

Figure 9.13   Contraceptive services – FP1002.

PART IV

DOCTOR'S CERTIFICATE AND CLAIM

FOR PAYMENT

To .... FAMILY PRACTITIONER COMMITTEE

(a) On .... (date) I fitted the person named overleaf with an intra-uterine device having had regard to and been guided by modern authoritative medical opinion such as the advice given in the Handbook of Contraceptive Practice issued by the Standing Medical Advisory Committee.

I claim the appropriate fee.

(b) Tick box
if
appropriate

☐   I previously accepted this patient for contraceptive services

in .... (date)

☐   The claim is made after the due date for renewal and I certify that services have been given continuously since that date. I apply for payment to be continuous.

	Name and address of doctor or partnership	For use by FPC

Signed ....

Date ....
(if different from (a) above)

SAMPLE

Printed in the UK for H.M.S.O. Dd8280533 C250 6/90 28312

Figure 9.13   *Continued*

NATIONAL HEALTH SERVICE   CONTRACEPTIVE SERVICES

TREATMENT OF PERSON TEMPORARILY ABSENT FROM HOME
PART 1
(to be completed by the patient)

Full forenames	Surname
Date of Birth	NHS Number (if known)
Present Address	
Home Address	
Name of doctor (if any) at home who has accepted me for contraceptive services	

I have received contraceptive services from the doctor whose signature appears below.

I am living for the time being at the Present Address shown above and do not expect to stay in the district more than 3 months from the date I was first given contraceptive services.

Date.. Signed...

(to be completed by the doctor)

I have given contraceptive services to the person named above having regard to and being guided by modern authoritative medical opinion such as the advice given in the Handbook of Contraceptive Practice issued by the Standing Medical Advisory Committee.

I claim the appropriate fee.

Date... Signed...

Name and address of doctor or partnership..

....

....

Form FP 1003

Figure 9.14   Contraceptive services – FP1003.

Record of treatment of temporary resident (FP19) (Figure 9.15)

This form is to be used to register a person who expects to be staying in the area for more than 24 hours but less than three months. Make sure the form is completed *in full* including if staying more than or less than 15 days. (There are two rates of fee paid – it is lower if the patient is staying less than 15 days.) The patient's signature is also required.

If the patient is requesting contraception, vaccination or maternity services *this form is not to be used.*

A *night visit* claim *can* be made if a temporary resident is visited at night.

Claims must be submitted within six months of the dated Temporary Resident form.

NATIONAL HEALTH SERVICE
**RECORD OF TREATMENT OF
TEMPORARY RESIDENT**

Cipher of Home FHSA

Surname	Mr Mrs Miss	NHS Number	Date of Birth

Forenames

Temporary
Address

Home
Address

Name of doctor at home

To be completed by patient

I am temporarily resident at the address shown above and I expect to remain in
the district for (tick whichever is appropriate)

not more than 15 days from today ☐

more than 15 days from today ☐

but not more than 3 months from the date of my arrival

I have received treatment from the doctor whose signature appears below.

Patient's signature ....

A person signing for the patient should state the relationship

To be completed by doctor

I have accepted the person named above as a Temporary Resident and have given
treatment which is not one of the exceptions listed in paragraph 32.12 of the
Statement of Fees and Allowances.

     * I also claim a rural Practice Payment. The distance from my main surgery

to the patient's temporary residence is ....miles.

Doctor's signature ....

Date...   Code No..
*Delete if not applicable.

Form FP 19 (Rev. 1992)

Figure 9.15   Record of treatment of temporary residents – FP19.

Claim in respect of emergency treatment (FP32)
(Figure 9.16)

The FP32 form is used if a patient who is not registered with the practice
attends for treatment and is not seeking acceptance but is unable to get to
their own GP or is a patient staying in the practice area for not more than
24 hours.

Form FP 32

NATIONAL HEALTH SERVICE

CLAIM IN RESPECT OF EMERGENCY TREATMENT

(For conditions see Statement of Fees and Allowances prepared by the Secretary of State—paragraphs 33.1–33.5)

SURNAME OF PATIENT ______ CHRISTIAN NAMES ______

HOME ADDRESS ______

ADDRESS AT TIME OF TREATMENT ______
(if different from above)

NATIONAL HEALTH SERVICE NO. ______

NAME OF PATIENT'S DOCTOR ______

PATIENT'S EXPLANATION OF NON-AVAILABILITY OF OWN DOCTOR OR HIS DEPUTY ______

DATE	TIME	†SERVICE RENDERED (Visit, Surgery attendance, etc.)	Place where service rendered	Fees
			If rural practice payment claimed enter distance	

Nature of accident or sudden emergency ______

Was the accident caused by, or did it arise out of, the use of a motor vehicle on a road? ______

I am informed that the patient was resident in the area for a period not exceeding 24 hours. (delete if not applicable).

Name of Claiming Doctor (in block Capitals) ______ Address ______

Signed ______ Code No. ______ Date ______

Claims should be made within 21 days of the date on which treatment was given.

†The nature of the service and the time and place at which it was rendered, should be shown in all claims

FOR OFFICE USE

1. Claim allowed / disallowed

2. Deduct / Do not deduct from patient's doctor

3. Initials

SAMPLE

Figure 9.16 Emergency treatment claim form – FP32.

Claim for immediately necessary treatment (FP106) (Figure 9.17)

The FP106 form is used if a patient who is not registered with the practice attends for treatment and the GP refuses to accept the patient on to his actual list or refuses to accept the patient as a temporary resident so long as the patient is not on the list of a GP in the area.

Arrest of dental haemorrhage (FP82)

A higher fee is paid for the arrest of a haemorrhage or the provision of after care. A lower fee is paid for the removal of plugs and stitches only (Figure 9.18).

FORM   FP 106

NAME OF PATIENT: SURNAME .... MR/MRS/MISS

                        FORENAMES ....

                        NHS. NO. ....

                        ADDRESS ....

                                 ....

TO BE COMPLETED BY THE PATIENT

I have today received treatment from the doctor whose signature appears below.
I have not been accepted for treatment by another doctor in the area or district.

PATIENT'S SIGNATURE ....

DATE   ....

TO BE COMPLETED BY THE DOCTOR

I have given immediately necessary treatment to the person named above.

    *   Whom I have refused to accept for inclusion on my list
        or as a temporary resident

    *   Who is to be assigned to me by the Secretary of State
        gives consent under regulation 14(1)

If treatment was limited to an item of service for which a fee is payable,
please indicate the nature of the service.

DOCTOR'S SIGNATURE   ....

DATE   ....   CODE NO. ....

* DELETE WHICHEVER IS INAPPLICABLE

FOR FAMILY PRACTITIONER COMMITTEE USE ONLY	NAME AND ADDRESS OF DOCTOR

Figure 9.17   Immediately necessary treatment claim form – FP106.

Remember

If treatment takes place at night you cannot claim a night visit fee *and* a fee for the dental haemorrhage. It is suggested a night visit fee is claimed as this is a higher fee.

Maternity medical services (FP24 (white) for GP on obstetric list otherwise FP24A (pink))

Each doctor should keep a book of maternity claims and as soon as pregnancy is confirmed get the patient to sign one. A completed claim form should show; date of booking, expected date of confinement (EDC), actual date of confinement and the date the patient left hospital (if you are claiming for full postnatal care).

It must be signed by the patient as soon as pregnancy is confirmed, and signed by the GP as soon as maternity care is complete (either: miscarriage, transfer to another GP or full postnatal examination). The form must be submitted to the FHSA within six months of the completion of services (Figure 9.19).

An antenatal care fee is paid when a patient is confined after the 24th week (or earlier if a live birth) even if the patient received all her antenatal care at a hospital. The fee decreases if the woman signs the maternity claim later in the pregnancy.

A miscarriage fee is paid if a pregnancy ends in a miscarriage before the end of 24th week. A fee cannot be claimed if the miscarriage occurred before the eighth week of pregnancy unless the patient had previously signed the claim form. (Please note: to avoid added distress a doctor can sign on the patient's behalf.)

If a GP helps during or just after labour he can claim a confinement fee even if the patient is not registered with him/her for maternity services.

To claim a complete maternity medical services fee the doctor has to offer antenatal care, care in confinement and postnatal care with a full postnatal examination within 12 weeks of delivery. Complete postnatal fees can be claimed if a GP supervises the delivery or the patient leaves hospital within 48 hours of delivery. Partial postnatal care can be claimed if the woman leaves hospital more than 48 hours after delivery. An extra fee can be claimed for up to five postnatal consultations/visits made within 14 days of delivery. A GP should perform a full postnatal examination 6 – 12 weeks after delivery.

To see how to complete the form FP24 see Figure 9.20.

NATIONAL HEALTH SERVICE

PART I (To be completed by the patient)

Surname of patient ....(Mr/Mrs/Miss)

Christian or forename(s) ....

Address ....

I received treatment from Dr. .... in connection with
the arrest of dental haemorrhage on ....

Delete if not (The treatment was given at my home in the course of a
appropriate   (visit by the doctor requested and made between the
              (hours of 10 pm and 8 am

....
Signature of patient (see note)

PART II (To be completed by the doctor)

I certify that I gave treatment for

    * the arrest of dental haemorrhage
    * the removal of dental plugs and/or dental stitches only

as indicated above and hereby apply for a fee of £ .... in
accordance with paragraph of the Statement of Fees and Allowances.

    * Delete if inappropriate

Date ....
                                        Signature of Doctor

PART III (For use by the Family Practitioner Committee)

┌─────────────────────────────────┐
│ Name and address of doctor: │
│   │
NOTE: A parent or guardian   │
       should sign on behalf   │
       of a child.   │
│   │
│   │
│   │
│   │
│   │
└─────────────────────────────────┘
                                     FP.82

Figure 9.18   Arrest of dental haemorrhage – FP82.

COUNTERFOIL.
(For Doctor's use)

NATIONAL HEALTH SERVICE   MATERNITY MEDICAL SERVICES

PART I

(to be detached and given to the patient)

Patient's name

To ....

I accept your application to receive maternity medical services from me.

E.D.C.

Your expected date of confinement is ....

Date ....   Doctor's signature ....

PART II

PATIENT'S APPLICATION FOR SERVICES

(Tick appropriate box)

Dr ....

A I wish to receive maternity medical services from you. I have not made arrangements for these services with another doctor. ☐

B I wish to receive maternity medical services from you. I have cancelled arrangements

made with Dr. ....

of .... ☐

Temporary resident

C I wish to receive maternity medical services from you whilst temporarily residing at:

....

.... ☐

Home doctor

I have made arrangements for maternity medical services in my home area with

Dr. ....

....

Emergency treatment

D I have received maternity medical services from you in an emergency. ☐

Patient's full name
(in block letters) ....

Home address

Home address ....

....

N.H.S. No.
or Date of Birth

Former name ....   N.H.S. No. ❶ ....
or Date of Birth

Date ....   Patient's signature ....

DOCTOR'S CERTIFICATE

(EMERGENCY ATTENDANCE FOR MISCARRIAGE)

Doctor's special certificate
(Miscarriage of
unbooked patient)

I certify that in the circumstances I thought it desirable, in the patient's interest, not to ask her for a signature.

Date ....   Doctor's signature ....

Form FP24

Figure 9.19   Maternity medical services claim form. FP24 for doctors included in 'obstetric list'. Doctors not included in list should use FP24A.

MATERNITY BENEFITS

There are cash benefits for mothers under the National Insurance Scheme which must be claimed within certain time limits. You are strongly advised to get Leaflet N.I. 17A and the necessary claim form from your local Maternity and Child Health Clinic, or from your local Department of Health and Social Security office not later than 14 weeks before your baby is expected.

PRESCRIPTION CHARGES AND WELFARE MILK AND VITAMINS

An expectant mother can apply on Part 1 of the Certificate of Pregnancy (Form FW8) for a prescription charge exemption certificate covering the period of her pregnancy and until her child is one year old. Details are given on Part 2 of Form FW8 and in leaflet MV11 (obtainable from Post Offices, local Department of Health and Social Security offices and local Maternity and Child Health Clinics) of how to claim free milk and vitamins.

PART III
DOCTOR'S CERTIFICATE AND CLAIM FOR PAYMENT
(References are to paragraphs in the Statement of Fees and Allowances)

(Tick appropriate box)

I certify that .... *(patient's name)*

(expected date of confinement .... **②** ......) had a miscarriage on ...... **③** ...... ☐ Miscarriage
                                                     was confined on .... ☐ Confinement

at home .... ☐ Home

In the GP Unit at .... **④** .... Hospital ☐

In .... Hospital ☐ Hospital

I further certify that I provided the services indicated below and that I had regard to and was guided by authoritative medical opinion as set out in paragraphs 31.2 and paragraph 31/Schedule 3.

Fees Claimed
(Paragraph 1/Schedule 1

(i) Complete Maternity Medical Services .... **⑤** .... Paras 31.7 to 31.8 ☐ Complete
(ii) Ante-natal care

Note: the date of booking is the date on which Parts I and II are completed

(a) Patient booked up to 16th week of pregnancy .... Para 31.9 ☐ Ante-natal
(b) Patient booked from 17th week to 30th week
    of pregnancy .... Para 31.9 ☐
(c) Patient booked from 31st week of pregnancy .... Para 31.9 ☐

(iii) Miscarriage .... **⑥** .... Para 31.10 ☐ Miscarriage
(iv) Care during the confinement .... Para 31.11 ☐ Confinement
(v) Complete Post-Natal Care (Date of Hospital Discharge ... **⑦** ...) Para 31.12 ☐ Complete post-natal
(vi) Partial Post-Natal Care .... Para 31.13 ☐ Partial post-natal
    (a) date of each attendance

    (b) date of full post-natal examination .... **⑧** ....
(vii) Other services as described in the attached note .... ☐ Other

(viii) Date of last service to patient ....
    (to be completed where only ante-natal care or only complete post-natal care is given).

I claim payment for the above services .... ☐

I also claim payment for the employment as anaesthetist of Dr. .... ☐
                                      Paras 31.15 to 31.16

Certificate to be signed
Date ....   Doctor's signature ....   in all cases.

Figure key:

1   enter correct NHS number
2   enter this date other than when claiming for post-natal care only
3   it is important that these dates are *clearly* entered as appropriate
4   please enter these sections correctly because different fees are payable
5   this section must be completed when complete care is provided
6   this section should be completed *only* when a woman has been confined at home or in a GP unit
7   this section should be completed *only* when a woman is confined in hospital (other than a GP unit) for less than 48 hours
8   this section should be completed when partial care is given.

Figure 9.19   *Continued*

MATERNITY MEDICAL SERVICES   FP24

Part 1:   to be addressed to pregnant patient giving date of expected confinement. Must be dated and signed by doctor. Then given to patient – this confirms in writing that GP is willing to give medical services

Part 11   to be completed by patient as soon as pregnancy confirmed–this confirms in writing that she wishes to receive maternity medical services

Part 111 to be completed after delivery before GP can submit claim

- an antenatal care fee can be claimed when a patient is confined after the 24th week (earlier if a live birth)

- there is a higher fee if the patient has signed the FP24 at 16 weeks or earlier; there is a lower fee paid if FP24 is signed from 31st week or later

- there is a fee paid if a miscarriage occurs before the end of the 24th week but after the 8th week

- even if a patient is not registered with GP but he has helped with delivery or immediately he (GP) can claim a confinement fee

- complete maternity medical services include antenatal care, care during the confinement and postnatal care which includes a full examination within 12 weeks of delivery

- if a GP supervises the delivery or the patient is discharged from hospital within 48 hours of delivery a confinement fee can be claimed

- if the patient is discharged more than 48 hours after delivery a GP can claim a partial postnatal care fee which includes an extra fee for up to five postnatal consultations made within the first 14 days of delivery

- a GP can claim a postnatal examination fee if a postnatal examination is performed six to twelve weeks after delivery.

Figure 9.20   How to complete FP24.

Dealing with patients who attend for treatment and who are not registered with the practice

Receptionists in general practice are often confronted with patients attending for treatment, but who are not registered with the practice. Confusion may occur as to which claim form should be completed so that the doctor may be paid a fee for his treatment. The following flow chart clearly illustrates when temporary resident fees (FP19), immediately necessary treatment fees (FP106), or emergency treatment fees (FP32) may be claimed. A patient, however, may wish to register with the practice, in which case forms FP4 or FP1 may be completed and the practice protocol for new patient registration followed (Figure 9.21).

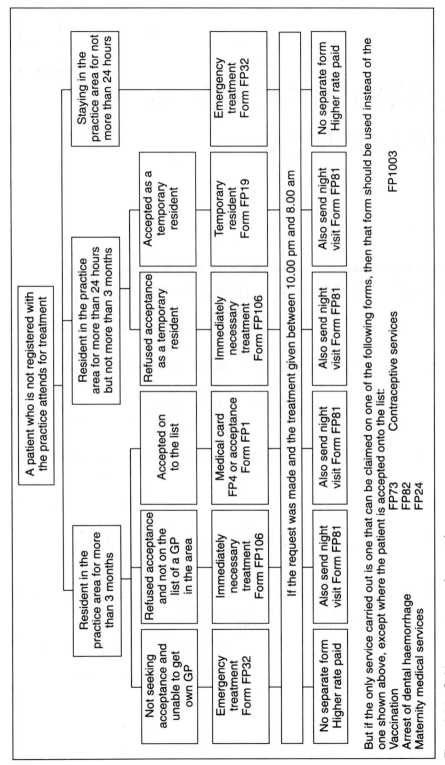

Figure 9.21   Guidance on usage of correct forms.

10

Using information technology

What's in the box – basic terminology

HARDWARE	Physical components of the system, such as display screens, printers, keyboard, mouse, discs, etc.
SOFTWARE	A set of programmed instructions in the computer which enable it to respond to input of information, and demands to change it, store it or print it out in various forms
CPU	The CPU, or central processor unit is the part of the system that performs arithmetic operations, and controls the storage, display, communication and manipulation of information. It is the part of the machine closest to a 'brain'
VDU	The screen used to display information held on the computer
KEYBOARD	A device like a typewriter to enter information into a computer. Many specialized systems use non-standard keyboards or make a lot of use of special function keys to save typing effort
MOUSE	A small hand operated pointer which the user moves on a pad to move an arrow on the screen. Clicking a button on the mouse activates a number of operations without the need to type in text

PRINTER	Prints text and diagrams held on the computer onto paper. Older machines work like typewriters and are noisy and slow. Newer types work more like photocopiers or paint sprayers, and are much faster and quieter
DISC	Information cannot be permanently stored in the CPU. Usually it is stored on magnetic disc or tape. Tape is used for long-term secure storage and disc for information in constant use
FLOPPY DISC	These are discs which can be inserted into one computer and read by another. Most are 3.5 inches in diameter and contained in a rigid plastic case
HARD DISC	These are permanently stored in the CPU and are used to store information needed on a permanent basis by a single user. Hard discs can hold many hundred times the information of a floppy
WORK STATION	The work area where a computer operator works. Health and safety legislation gives details of how work stations should be designed
TERMINAL	A machine capable of entering and retrieving information from a multi-user computer system. It may be a computer in its own right or, more usually, just a keyboard and screen
NETWORK	When many people need to use the same computer system, several terminals can be linked together with cables. This, and the software needed for communication with a central CPU, is called a network
BYTE	This is the measure of information a computer can store. A byte is equivalent to a single text character, one megabyte equals one million bytes. The more bytes of memory a computer, or disc, has, the more information it can store

How a computer works

It is not necessary to understand fully how computers work in order to operate the systems in use in GP practices, clinics and hospitals. The following brief outline is given for interest.

The central processor unit uses a system of on–off switches to hold information in a memory. Each number or character is expressed as a sequence of on or off states in a group of switches which together form a *byte*. As the operator enters information into the computer it is translated into machine readable form and stored in the *random access memory* (RAM). This process is controlled by the computer's internal *operating system*. This is the raw material which is worked on by the computer's *application software*, which tells the machine how to display and manipulate the data to achieve the operator's needs and how to interpret the instructions given by the operator.

The most common types of software are *word processors* which enable users to write documents, edit and print them. Most have facilities to store lists of names and addresses and write these into one of a series of previously written standard letters. Routine correspondence can be produced far more efficiently in this way. Individual parts of a document can be edited without the need for wholesale retyping. Importantly, information stored on one computer within a system (such as a patient administration system), can be imported onto another without the need to retype it.

Databases are applications designed to hold a lot of information about a series of people or things. An individual record (a patient for instance) contains a variety of *fields* which may have general text such as name, address and details of medical conditions. The field could have a specialized or limited range of values like a postcode, date, male or female; or it could be a code obtained from a published table like diagnostic codings for different medical conditions. These codes are much easier for a computer system to analyse than free text which really needs a human brain to interpret.

Spreadsheets are especially suited to putting in order, displaying and performing calculations on mathematical data. They are commonly used to analyse treatments given to a large number of patients or to calculate and report on budgets and expenditure. A typical small spreadsheet is shown below:

PROJECTED QUARTERLY EXPENDITURE ON STAFF TRAINING				
Expenditure	First quarter	Second quarter	Third quarter	Fourth quarter
Staff time	£1287	£10 663	£7287	£5288
Expenses	£325	£8825	£8350	£3000
Total	£1612	£19 488	£15 637	£8288

Computers in general practice

General practice today is such a complex organization, and it is doubtful whether management of its administration can be effectively handled without information technology (IT). A computerized practice is:

- more efficient
- in greater control of patient care
- able to generate more income.

Patient benefits through computerization

- Improved preventive care through the identification of 'at risk' groups, patient group analysis and follow-up.
- Reducing the risk of disease through immunization/vaccination.
- The early detection of disease through developmental screening, hypertensive monitoring, geriatric surveillance, etc.
- The management of established disease.
- More selective advice on smoking, drinking, etc.
- Better information on the patient services available.*

*(Source: Royal College of General Practitioners, *Computers in General Practice Guidance Notes*.)

The uses of an up-to-date patient database include:

- patient information data
- age – sex register
- logging and generation of repeat prescriptions
- logging and checking patient registration status
- checking immunization/cervical cytology status
- screening and recall
- diagnosis and morbidity data
- opportunistic screening.

A computerized appointments system overcomes the difficulties of manual appointment books, e.g. illegible handwriting, pages messy with cancellations, two people not being able to use the book at the same time, handwritten surgery lists for pulling out records, are all circumvented.

Reference had been made to using IT for written communication in Chapter 3. Secretaries and receptionists are now able to produce letters using a wordprocessing package to generate mail-merged letters, or readily produce letters to patients. Spreadsheets can be used either to collect data (for display in tables, graphs and pie charts) or to present doctor and staff rotas.

Desktop publishing software can be used to generate leaflets, posters and handouts.

Technology can save time for some tasks; in others it does not save time, but it does make it possible to produce professional looking documents, for example, practice leaflets, charts and posters.

For those who enjoy using a computer, it is essential that the computer does not become an obstacle between the patient and the secretary or receptionist. Remember, it is equally rude to continue to input/extract data as it is to continue to talk to a colleague or take a telephone call without acknowledging the presence of a patient.

The major disadvantage of IT in the practice is when the system 'goes down'; the increased efficiency disappears and returning to manual systems, no matter how temporarily, results in unavoidable delays and disruption.

Age–sex register and patient information

These are basic patient data put on to the computer. Secretaries and receptionists will receive specific training in the use of their practice's information system.

The importance of inputting data accurately cannot be overstated as this information will be of vital importance to the practice's activities. Remember, too, to always input the postcode; it is a vital piece of information and should be cross checked with the medical record in your possession.

You should be aware of the requirements of the Data Protection Act, and must respect the security and confidentiality of patient information at all times.

Registration data

This information is of immense value; it includes all information regarding registration status:

- date patient registered with the practice
- date patient was accepted on the doctor's list
- date patient was included in a GP's patient list.

It will also indicate the category and date of a patient's removal from a doctor's list, e.g., when moving out of the area, or on death.

Repeat prescriptions

A computerized system can save much of the receptionist's time by obviating the need to retrieve patient files and other manually held prescribing information. It also:

- produces a legible, printed and accurate prescription
- places a time limit on the issue of repeat prescriptions
- monitors the rate and consumption of drugs
- updates the repeat prescription record
- identifies easily patients who are on a particular medication.

Screening and recall

The ability of a computer to search rapidly on specific criteria can allow a practice to identify certain groups of patients:

- selected for information (e.g. asthmatics, hypertensives, diabetics, etc.) for health promotion banding, and who would benefit from additional care and those who are considered to be 'at risk'
- who are eligible for item-of-service claims.

The computer can also help with:

- crisis intervention
- the control of chronic diseases
- preventive medicine
- generating additional income for the practice.

Diagnoses and morbidity

A computer has the capacity and speed to extract and analyse data on any topics of particular interest to the practice, for example to analyse morbidity and treatment within the practice. The latest RCGP (Royal College of General Practitioners) coding system has been developed with a view to collecting these type of data from as many practices as possible.

Social recording

Computer systems are also capable of recording information on height/weight/smoking and alcohol habits so as to provide the FHSA with statistics for practices claiming health promotion banding allowances. This information is automatically included in the patients' records.

Computers in hospitals

Computerization of records in a hospital works well because there is a great deal of information to be stored and consulted, information is required by a variety of people at different times and in different locations, much of the information needs to be sorted or changed and complex analysis of data is needed.

This is not because computers are 'clever'. They are not, they have no real intelligence or ability to think of solutions. However computers can process vast amounts of data at incredible speed with virtually no errors. A 'computer error' is almost always a human operator doing the wrong thing or the computer's programmer setting it up wrongly in the first place.

The main systems used in hospitals are the patient administration system (PAS), word processing, and record storage in pathology, X-ray and pharmacy. Other major systems are used in finance and personnel departments, estates management and supplies, and are being introduced into nursing and theatre management.

Patient administration systems (PAS)

The potential of computers has long been exploited in hospitals in the area of patient administration. There are many versions used by different hospitals, but all have the following component parts:

PATIENT INDEX	Records of the personal details of every patient
ADMISSIONS, DISCHARGES AND TRANSFERS	A record of each patient's history of time spent in the hospital as an inpatient or outpatient, with particular consultants or in a particular department
WAITING LISTS	Names and dates of referral of all patients waiting for inpatient and/or outpatient treatment
OUTPATIENTS	A system to manage appointments and correspondence associated with outpatient clinics
GP INDEX	A list of the names and addresses of all the local GPs

Nursing management systems

Increasingly, hospitals are being equipped with computer systems to help nurses plan and keep track of the nursing care of patients. Patients' details are retrieved from PAS and a detailed plan of their expected care is prepared. Care given is recorded onto the system to help co-ordinate the work of the team. Patient dependency levels can be predicted from the care plans and nurse rosters are drawn up to match needs.

Order communication systems

In most hospitals, ordering portering services, pathology tests, supplies of materials or repairs to buildings or equipment must be done by telephone or by completing a form, often with multiple copies and posting it to the relevant department. This can take a long time and involve much duplication of effort. An order communications (or 'order-comms') system allows ordering departments to send requests for services directly to the department, and receive confirmation of orders or the results of tests directly.

Hospital information support system (HISS)

The trend among hospitals with well established computer systems is to integrate them into one powerful scheme called a hospital information support system (HISS). Such a system allows every department's computer system to talk to those of other departments, to transfer information and to generate reports.

Getting the best from the computer

The importance of inputting data accurately cannot be overstated, as this information is to be used by health care professionals in treating and caring for patients, for statistical analysis and planning, for budgeting, for contract monitoring and invoicing for services. Information held on the computer must be regularly cross-checked with that held on medical records, and amended as necessary. Incorrect information about a patient can lead to important letters or test results going astray.

Frequent problems which arise in hospitals are caused by out-of-date addresses, either because the patient has moved house or changed GP or both. Other problems arise from incomplete details, or temporary addresses entered as permanent, for example when a person is taken ill when visiting relatives. Errors in this information can be very costly to the hospital, since if the bill is sent to the wrong health authority or GP fund-holder they are unlikely to pay.

The barrier created by the computer

Computer systems usually require patient information to be input in a specific sequence which may not be the same as that which the patient wants to give. Sometimes the computer is slow to respond if a lot of people are using it. Receptionist staff frequently have to deal with a patient on the phone, another in person and call up details onto their screen, all at the same time. Both patient and receptionist start to feel that they are the servant of the computer, rather than the other way round.

To overcome these difficulties it is important to explain to the patient what is happening (especially when on the telephone) and develop a sequence of questions which gives the information you need in the correct order. This often requires a good deal of practice and discussion with colleagues before it works really well.

Maintaining security

There are four main risks to be guarded against when using computer systems:

• unauthorized access to information held on computer

- loss of information due to mechanical failure
- theft of machinery
- spoiling of information by computer viruses.

Preventing unauthorized access

Information about people held on computer is governed by the Data Protection Act. It should only be used for the purpose for which it was collected and should not be revealed to unauthorized people. Where password systems exist, these must be used. Passwords should never be shared or revealed to others. Computer screens should face away from public areas. Terminals should not be left unattended showing data or even 'logged in' to a system, since anyone may then gain access.

Backing up – keeping spare copies of information

If information has been stored on a computer's hard disc and it is lost due to mechanical failure or theft a great deal of work will be needed to replace it. It is extremely important to keep copies on a separate storage device. Taking such copies is known as backing up and should be done daily. Staff using a multi-user system may find that it is done centrally by a system manager. Each night the latest data is copied on to large tape recorders.

Personal computers should be backed up either to a central back up store via a hospital network, or to removable floppy discs, or specially designed tape records (called tape streamers). Locally made back up copies should be stored away from the computer in case of theft or fire.

Guarding against theft

Backing up is also important in case a computer is stolen. Such thefts are becoming increasingly common from hospitals and health care premises. Premises should be secure and kept locked. Machinery should be indelibly marked and preferably fastened to the desktop and alarmed with one of a variety of proprietary products. Computers should be housed away from public view wherever possible, e.g. away from windows without blinds.

Computer viruses

These are small programs designed to damage data held on computer. They are transferred from one machine to another when other files are copied, perhaps from floppy disc or by electronic connection. To guard against this, material should never be copied from a disc which has not been checked for viruses, nor should games and other such programs be copied onto work machines. Computer equipment and discs should be routinely checked for the presence of virus programs.

Illegal use of software

Commercial computer programs are protected by copyright. Generally a program can only be used on one computer unless a site licence has been purchased. The penalties for using programs which are not licensed are extremely high.

Computers and the law

Where medical records are stored on computer it is a requirement that computer-held material is at least as confidential as a paper record. Special care must be taken with computerized information, since it is possible to write programs which allow different people different levels of access. For example, it is possible to give a doctor access via the computer to all the information held, whereas the clerk may only see certain material. Some staff will be allowed to change information, others will have 'read only' access

The Data Protection Act 1984 (see Chapter 4)

Organizations which record information relating to identifiable living individuals on computer must ensure that they comply with the provisions of the Data Protection Act. This Act applies to England, Wales, Scotland and Northern Ireland.

The Data Protection Act is based on eight principles and is designed to ensure that information relating to an individual is obtained fairly, is kept up to date and is stored securely. The individual whose data are stored has rights of access enabling him or her to check the accuracy of the information. The data protection registrar and the courts are empowered to require correction of inaccurate material if it is not undertaken voluntarily by the data user.

Looking ahead

Information technology is rapidly advancing, and many medical practices are linked directly to health authorities. As a result many procedures are changing, for example: all new patient registrations will be carried out by computer and all night visits will be computerized.

11

Medical terminology and clinical aspects

Introduction

Medical secretaries and receptionists, with their unique skills of dealing with doctors, other professionals and patients, with tact and courtesy, will find that a knowledge of medical terminology will help them to carry out their duties in a more effective and efficient manner. Very often the words and phrases used by medical professionals are long, difficult and frequently appear to be obscure.

Medical terminology is based upon root words derived from Greek and Latin. To these roots may be added syllabi that modify the meaning of the root word. An addition made to the front of a root is known as a *prefix;* an addition at the end is a *suffix.* Over the years this principle has been modified in such a way that it can be applied to modern medical techniques. For example, the root 'gaster' means 'stomach'. By adding the suffix 'itis' the word is modified to mean 'inflammation of the stomach'; or by the addition of 'oscopy' we have gastroscopy, which means in this modified form 'visual inspection of the stomach' (by means of a gastroscope).

It is not intended to go into a detailed explanation of medical terminology, but to point out that a limited knowledge of some root words, prefixes and suffixes will give a wider understanding of the medical vocabulary. Appendix 4 lists some of the most commonly used root words, prefixes and suffixes.

Medical abbreviations are also frequently used by professionals in health care, and a knowledge of these will also be of value. (See Appendix 4.)

Pathology and X-ray examinations

Medical secretaries and receptionists will find that doctors refer patients for pathological and other investigations and tests. An awareness of the most commonly used tests will not only contribute to the effectiveness of their day-to-day work, but will also make their job more interesting and fulfilling. (See Appendix 4.)

Prescribing and drugs

The supply, distribution and storage of drugs are controlled by a series of Acts of Parliament, designed to control their sale and to reduce their danger to life from sale by unqualified persons.

Secretaries and receptionists will find that a knowledge of the drugs most frequently used by the medical practice or hospital consultant will be of value in their day-to-day work.

Receptionists in general practice have greater direct involvement with repeat prescribing for their patients and will often have to deal with queries. However, the receptionist must have clear instructions and never be placed in the position of making medical decisions.

Components of a prescription

The following information must be included on every prescription issued by the doctor, whether it be an NHS or a private prescription. Without this information it is not possible for the pharmacist to dispense the drugs. Sometimes it could be that the writing on the prescription is illegible, but this is not so common now that repeat prescriptions in general practice are computer-generated.

Drug name

This may be written in the generic or approved name of the drug, or its trade, or proprietary name (see also page 197). For example:

- salbutamol (generic)
- Ventolin (proprietary).

Form of prescribed drug

This refers to whether capsules, tablets, syrup, injection, ointment, etc. are required.

Strength

Many drugs are available in more than one strength, which must be specified.

Directions

Directions to the patient regarding dosage of the medicine should be included. The *British National Formulary* recommends that directions should preferably be in English. Some doctors still use Latin abbreviations. (See Appendix 4.)

Amount or quantity

A box on the prescription form can be completed to indicate the number of days treatment is to continue. If this is not used, the quantity to be dispensed should be included.

Problems from prescriptions

Medical receptionists and secretaries should be aware that problems can be caused by:

- missing information, e.g. strength of drug, missing form or type of drug, missing dose
- incorrect or inaccurate information, e.g. incorrect name of drug (similar drug names can cause problems – *chlorpropamide* which is used for diabetics and *chlorpromazine*, a tranquillizer)
- incorrect strength or incorrect dose
- amounts of medicine prescribed (patients often complain that they have run out of one medicine and still have some others left. Remember, medicines come in different pack sizes – some in 28s some in 30s, etc.)

Controlled drugs

The relevant legislation concerning controlled drugs is the Misuse of Drugs Regulations 1985 and subsequent amendments.

For controlled drugs there are rules for :

- who can possess and supply
- record keeping
- storage
- prescription writing.

Records

Secretaries and receptionists should understand that it is the doctor's duty to maintain a register, in an approved form, of the quantity of all controlled drugs obtained and supplied, including any administered personally, including names and addresses.

Storage

All controlled drugs in the custody of a doctor, must be kept in a locked cupboard that can only be opened by the doctor or with his/her authority.

It is the doctor's responsibility to ensure the controlled drugs cupboard is locked and the keys put safely away. The medical secretary or receptionist should make sure that this has been done.

Prescribing controlled drugs

Special rules apply to prescribing controlled drugs. A prescription for a controlled drug must:

- be written in ink, or otherwise so as to be indelible; it must be signed and dated by the person issuing it with his/her usual signature
- be written by the person issuing it in their own handwriting
- specify the name and address of the person for whom it is intended
- specify the strength of the preparation, the dose to be taken and the quantity of the preparation in both words and figures.

An exception to these rules is for phenobarbitone – receptionists can write these prescriptions, but the quantity must be written in both words and figures.

Repeat prescribing

The doctor is responsible for issuing the initial prescription to the patient, and explaining what the preparation is and what it is intended to do, etc. The patient does not always remember and will often discuss any problems with the receptionist or secretary.

Some patients are on regular drug regimes and are able to request repeat prescriptions without seeing the doctor every time they run out of their medication.

In general practice, receptionists play a vital role in the repeat prescription procedure of the practice:

- They receive the requests from patients for a repeat of their medication.

- They will either prepare a further prescription for the doctor's signature, or generate a repeat prescription on the practice computer to be signed by the doctor.

- A record should be kept either on the computer or in the patient's medical record (or both) of repeat prescribing.

- They will explain to the patient how to make the best use of the repeat prescription service offered by the practice, for example, the procedures and system used – the use of cards, computer print-out, or telephone requests for repeat prescriptions.

The repeat prescription system used by the medical practice is designed not only to make better use of the doctor's time, but to suit the patient's needs. Every practice has its own system to ensure that patients get their prescriptions on a regular basis.

Computer-generated prescriptions

Many practices now have a computer which will generate repeat prescriptions, instead of receptionists laboriously writing them out. Although computer-generated prescriptions are time saving, secretaries and receptionists must remember that computers are only efficient if the correct information has been entered in the first instance. Therefore, when entering details of patients' medication into the computer, always check that all the information is there, for example, the right drug, its strength, the correct dose and quantity have been entered.

Sources of information

Doctors receive a great deal of information which is designed to help them in prescribing for their patients. Medical secretaries and receptionists will, no doubt, have access to the following useful sources of information:

- *British National Formulary (BNF)*
- *Monthly Index of Medical Specialities (MIMS)*.

The BNF, published twice yearly, is an official reliable source of accurate information on prescribing. MIMS is sent to doctors each month. It is a good, 'user-friendly' information source, but printing errors may occasionally occur. Both publications provide details of constituents, manufacturers, packaging, net costs, etc. of every medicine that can be prescribed.

Branded or generic

Every drug that a doctor prescribes will fall into one of two categories:

- branded
- generic.

The term 'branded' refers to the proprietary name of a drug given by a manufacturer, whilst, 'generic' means that the name is a general one which describes the pharmacological product. Both the *BNF* and *MIMS* give cross-referenced information on generic and brand-named products.

Practice prescribing policies

Prescription analysis and cost (PACT)

Secretaries and receptionists in general practice will be aware that their practice prescribing policy reflects, to a certain extent, national and local guidelines.

The Prescription Pricing Authority (PPA) sends a statement each quarter giving information on what individual doctors, and the whole practice is prescribing, how much is being spent on drugs, and how they compare locally and nationally with other doctors and practices. Health authorities indicate a target cost for each practice to aim for, which is designed to encourage effective prescribing procedures.

Practice formularies

There are many medicines and preparations available on preschool, a number of which are the same generic drug with a different proprietary name. Practices are reducing the number of drugs they prescribe, and where appropriate, yet in the patients' best interests, will try to achieve the national approach.

The community pharmacist

Pharmacists, in common with general practitioners, have a contract with the NHS, which clearly states their terms of service. This contract, together with the requirements of the Medicines Act, provides the framework in which pharmacists work.

The pharmacist is a professional person who will, from time to time telephone a medical practice to speak to a doctor, or member of the team. This may be to query a prescription item or the frequency of its repeat. The receptionist or secretary should always immediately connect the pharmacist to the doctor, being aware that they are acting in accordance with legal and professional responsibility.

Many community pharmacists keep computerized records of medicines dispensed to patients, and are thus readily aware of potential problems.

12

Primary health care services and social services

Introduction

The government's policy in recent years has been to transfer care from the secondary to the primary sector, i.e. from hospitals or other institutions (such as long-term inpatient psychiatric care), to the patients being at home and supported there by relevant services.

These policies are embodied in the Health of the Nation documents which set out health targets for the nation. Within local settings, for example in Wales, health authorities and FHSAs/health boards have set out local strategies for health aligned with the Health of the Nation strategy, but breaking it down into achievable aims and objectives at the local level. The Community Care Act supplements the Health of the Nation strategy by providing a structure to manage the patients in their homes.

The Community Care Act gives patients (or clients) an active part in deciding what care they receive, compared to the previous situation where the health authority and social services provided a range of services and the patient received the service deemed most appropriate by doctors, nurses or social workers.

Care in the community includes both community nursing services and social services. As each patient is referred to the community nursing services (either from a hospital, a general practitioner or by self referral) an assessment is carried out with the patient, and their relatives if they wish, in the home. A nursing care plan is agreed which is tailored to meet the needs of the patient. Typical services provided by community nurses would include giving injections, e.g. insulin to housebound diabetics, palliative care to patients who are dying, dressings and removal of stitches after surgery. Patients do not make any personal contribution to the cost of their care, i.e. the service is free.

With social services, a care plan is agreed between the patient and the social worker, however, the patient's financial situation is also taken into account to work out the patient's contribution towards cost. (Patients have made a contribution towards social services received for some time and no one goes without a service they need simply because they cannot afford it.) Social services provide for children and families, the elderly, patients with mental illness, learning difficulties, permanent disabilities and alcohol problems. To supplement care given by families, friends and neighbours, help may come from:

- social workers, home carers, meals on wheels
- sheltered housing, day centres, residential homes, nursing homes
- wardens and housing officers
- voluntary groups, visitors and churches.

Apart from meals on wheels which delivers a hot cooked meal to the patient's home, luncheon clubs encourage patients to socialize, carer support groups encourage family members and friends to share their experiences and support one another, and information services help patients and families to know what is available to them. Simple practical help, such as assistance with bathing, light housework, or preparing a meal is now provided by home carers who are specially trained to do this work.

Further information about community nursing or social services provided in any particular area of the country will be available from local offices who publish leaflets outlining what they provide, to whom and how to access the services.

The limit on funds for health and social care results in decisions being made about what service or care is received dependent on money available. This concept is very difficult for a nation that has come to depend on a free health service available to all at the point of need. The reality of the situation is that the government does not have a bottomless purse, so the responsibility for deciding who receives what care is being transferred to those who deal with the patients – doctors, health and social care workers. Therefore the role of health professionals is changing from 'helping people' and responding to need, to include assessment and management, and offsetting need against available funds.

Dentists, opticians and pharmacists, like general practitioners, are contracted to the FHSAs to provide their services. They are also greatly affected by the changes to the funding and structure of the health service. Fewer dental and optical services are available to patients on the NHS so their NHS income has dropped. To remain viable they charge patients for services and sell related products, or become entirely private practice. Pharmacists' income is directly related to the value of prescriptions dispensed. Doctors are reducing their prescription bills to meet their indicative prescribing budgets and so pharmacists' income is also dropping. They supplement their income by selling more 'over the counter' and associated products and some independent local chemists are being taken over by larger chains.

Fundholding and trust status

General practitioners have been offered the opportunity to become fundholders, which allows them to contract with hospitals for investigations (X-rays, blood tests, etc.) and some inpatient and outpatient referrals. Emergency admissions, children, maternity, the elderly and some specialities (e.g. renal dialysis) are not included in the fundholding budgets at this time. There are also budgets for prescribing, staff and fund management. The administration of the funds (or budgets) is a paper exercise since the practices do not actually receive the money. They raise invoices for patient services and authorize payment to the trust hospitals via the FHSA when notification of the care given to each patient is returned to the surgery. Trust hospitals are those which choose to manage their own budgets; they apply for and attain trust status, so that they can contract to provide specific services to general practice.

Where a practice negotiates contracts including clauses, for example, where their patients will be seen within six weeks of referral, and admitted with a further four weeks, it becomes clear that patients of fundholding practices are seen more quickly. The government has therefore laid down conditions to ensure that patients of non-fundholding practices do not have to be on a waiting list longer than one year. This is a considerable improvement on waiting lists where, for a few specialities in some areas of the country, about five years ago a wait of well over two years was not unknown.

The change from institutionalization to locally managed units is such a complex one that the government has phased the introduction allowing keen well-organized practices to be in the first wave in 1990. Subsequent years have been referred to as second, third and fourth waves. The health authority, through district management units, ensures provision of the services not covered by fundholding. Similarly they provide services for practices and hospitals either not included, or who do not wish to be included, in the fundholding/trust system.

Despite new problems generated from the changes, trust status hospitals provide the service that practitioners now demand so this should benefit the majority of patients immediately and ultimately all patients.

Trust status has also been given to ambulance services. Their whole range of services from transporting patients to hospital outpatient clinics, emergency admissions, doctors' answering service, paging, community alarms and nursing answering service are now managed against budgets with built-in standards of achievement, e.g. for patients being transported to a particular clinic, they will be picked up and returned within a specific time of their appointment so that they are not kept waiting around the hospital for hours on end.

The patient and the receptionist

From the patient's view there are no major changes to services, since they are all still available, but should be more efficient as they are delivered according to Patients' Charters. A Patients' Charter is a document setting out the standard of service to be provided in layman's language.

Receptionists arranging access to services will find that procedures depend on local arrangements, i.e. whether the particular service has gained trust status or whether it is still under the management of the health authority. Set procedures can only be specified by referring to the local offices of the ambulance service, social or community services. It is advisable for staff responsible for arranging transport to visit ambulance headquarters to see at first hand how requests for transport are processed.

As a result of the primary health care sector growing, the role of the receptionist, clerical and secretarial staff, both in the hospital and in general practice, is becoming increasingly complex as the changes are effected. No longer do staff merely 'go between' the doctor and patient, but must now liaise with hospital departments, community and social services. Every few months another department or service moves, changes its name, and its personnel change their function or role. It is important for all staff to understand the difficulties experienced in other sectors of health and social care provision as they cope with the fundamental changes going on around them.

Although doctors' surgery staff may have been recognized as part of the primary health care team for some time, their importance as key members in providing a communication link is growing with the size of the team and the increased variety of necessary points of contact. Similarly, surgery and hospital staff need to be aware of their new role as the government puts greater emphasis onto health promotion.

The primary health care team

The change of emphasis from institutionalized health care provision to management by smaller sections within the services generates a greater need for deliberate integration of the various services so that patients are presented with 'seamless' health and social care.

Staff increasingly become involed in dealing with queries, passing messages, and ensuring that the patients released from long-term institutionalized care, or fresh from surgical procedures, receive the service they need from the various members of the extended primary health care team.

From the 1960s, as health authorities built health centres, accommodation was provided for the community, social and other services, including chiropody, dental and dispensaries. This made it easier for doctors and receptionists to communicate with, for example, community staff, because they were likely to meet in the health centre. In the last few years there has been a general move to 'attach' community staff to specific surgeries where the premises are privately owned by the doctors. A message book is kept in reception so that messages can be picked up easily, and office space is made available.

The benefits of better communication have been supplemented by developing primary health care team meetings. These may have a strong clinical flavour, where doctors and health visitors, midwives, and social workers discuss the needs of specific patients. Alternatively, meetings where strategies are developed for defining and maintaining management and administration of the team would also include reception and administration staff. It is essential to have a chair person to control the agenda so that the subject areas are of interest to everyone. Even if meetings are only held monthly, getting together a group of up to 40 people on a regular basis can be extremely difficult. It is important, therefore, to produce brief minutes so that those who are unable to attend can follow up issues with colleagues.

The primary health care team in its broadest sense includes doctors, practice nurses, the practice manager, reception and administration staff, health visitors, midwives, community nursing stafff, social workers, community psychiatric nurses and any other nursing specialists. Within this team, however, there are other teams, e.g. receptionists, practice nurses, practice, community and psychiatric nurses, and so on. Each team should work together for the common good, so it is important for each member to appreciate the role and purpose of the other members.

The general medical practitioner

The GP is at the centre of primary health care. The doctor's surgery represents the entrance to most of the services provided by the NHS and the GP's responsibility is to maintain the health of patients and their families by treatment, prevention and health education. GPs give personal and continuing care to their patients, and are in a position to build up a relationship of trust. They attend patients in their consulting room and in their homes. The GP aims to make initial diagnoses of problems presented, to provide treatment as appropriate, or where necessary to refer patients for further professional treatment.

The practice manager

The practice manager is the person to whom both secretaries and receptionists in general practice are accountable. He/she has a central role in the day-to-day smooth running of the practice to ensure a quality service to the patients. The manager is the leader responsible for building, maintaining and co-ordinating the practice team so that the objectives are achieved and tasks completed satisfactorily. The manager also has the responsibility of developing and training individuals and helping them to realize their potential. They are the person secretaries and receptionists will go to to discuss any difficulties and problems experienced in the workplace.

Community nursing sisters

These used to be known as district nurses because they worked on a geographical basis looking after the nursing needs of patients in their own homes. They are now more often than not attached to a single practice and work with the patients belonging to that practice, or perhaps the patients of two smaller practices. Practice attachment gives them a chance to work more closely in a team with other staff but has the disadvantage of spreading their work over a very wide area. Occasionally these nurses work in the treatment room of the practice. They are employed by the health authority and are fully trained nurses who have experience in hospitals before coming to work in the community. They are involved in traditional nursing duties such as treating people who are ill at home with heart failure, acute chest conditions, terminal illness or, increasingly, after early discharge from hospital. These patients may require wound dressings, attention to bowels, prevention of bed sores and so on, and their relatives at home will gain great support from being taught how to help the patients themselves or just by knowing that someone will be coming in regularly.

Health visitors

The health visitor is a trained nurse with a post-registration qualification, employed by the District Health Authority, and working mainly as a member of the primary health care team. The training of health visitors is rooted in the promotion of health and they learn to recognize the effects of psychological, social, economic and environmental factors on health and this enables them to fulfil their role in health education and the prevention of disease.

Although health visitors are concerned with all age groups, they have a special responsibility for the under-fives. New-born babies are visited in their own homes, and parents advised on matters of child health and development. Emphasis is given to the need for immunization and the value of attending a child health clinic. They are also concerned with other vulnerable groups such as the elderly, the physically and mentally handicapped, single parents, and families under stress. In addition they may be involved in the provision of health surveillance programmes and research, in which case an age-sex register or other form of database is particularly helpful.

Practice nurses

These form a rapidly growing group of health care workers and represent one way by which health services are changing to meet new challenges. They are usually employed by the practice and do most of their work within the treatment room. They are usually fully trained nurses who have had experience in hospital and other fields before taking up practice work. Practice nurses are employed in traditional work in the treament room such as applying dressings, giving injections, syringing ears and removing sutures. The range of their activity is changing to include helping to run health promotion clinics, assist with child health surveillance and minor surgery. They are thus often specially trained in the management of chronic illness such as asthma, diabetes and hypertension. Practice nurses are beginning to use some of the tools that were traditionally used only by the doctor such as ophthalmoscopes, stethoscopes, auroscopes and vaginal speculae. Further important extensions of their work involve counselling, listening and reassuring.

Midwives

Midwives have a central role in the care of pregnant women. They are fully trained nurses who have then completed a prolonged midwifery course. They are employed by the health authority and they form part of the team with hospital obstetricians, general practitioners and health visitors concerned with antenatal care, antenatal preparation, intrapartum care, delivery, and postpartum care of the mother and infant. They run antenatal clinics sometimes with doctors, and conduct normal deliveries in hospital and occasionally in the home. They are also very much involved in the postpartum care of mothers discharged home early after delivery.

Social workers

In about one in five consultations a doctor becomes involved in discussions and advice about personal relationships, work, social benefits, social support or other financial matters. These are important features of primary care, but just as the doctor will want to call on the special skills of nurses for some problems, so he will want to use a social worker's skills in the issues listed above.

If, for example, a young single mother is taken ill the problem extends beyond the immediate care of a sick woman and involves a healthy child also. If an elderly person living alone has a minor stroke which limits their independence by making it difficult to cook, clean or shop, another sort of problem arises that might best be solved by a home help, meals on wheels or laundry services. The social worker will help in assessing the need for this service, and in setting up these forms of care if they are needed. Again, if family tensions threaten dangers to the wife or children, supervision and counselling may be required and is most likely to be dealt with by a social worker.

There are some specialized social workers – these include psychiatric social workers who are important in the involuntary admission of the psychiatrically sick and in helping and supporting the long-term sick such as patients who are schizophrenics, or those with senile dementia who live in the community.

Community psychiatric nurses

Community psychiatric nurses belong to a profession which, although still in its infancy, is of increasing importance. Their role has developed with the trend towards rehabilitating and caring for the mentally infirm in the community. Although they may be used in psychiatric hospitals they are largely involved in providing support and treatment in collaboration with general practitioners. They tend to act as independant clinical practitioners themselves, backed by both consultants and general practitioners, with the object of restricting long-term hospital treatment to the severest cases only.

Pharmacists

We see in another section how doctors and pharmacists relate to each other in terms of their activities with prescriptions. Many patients go first to the pharmacist with their complaint and may never need to see the doctor. Others are advised by the pharmacist that a consultation is necessary. Communication between the two professions is very important.

Home helps

Home helps play a vital role in keeping the elderly in their homes for as long as possible. Their role is to perform those domestic tasks – such as shopping, washing, cleaning and collecting pensions – which the elderly can no longer undertake because of infirmity. They have no clinical responsibility but their visits provide a friendly and caring link with the outside world. It is usually the social services department of the local authority that organizes their work.

Other members

There is a large variety of other skilled workers who, from time to time, become part of the team. Experts like chiropodists, dietitians, physiotherapists, clinical psychologists, pharmacists and so on, may be involved.

The principal skill of clinical psychologists is in the realm of personal development and interpersonal relationship. They can help with behavioural problems of children and teenagers, getting people to cope with life's difficulties, marital problems and so on.

Home care teams

We have seen that some teams consist of people employed by the practice, whilst others consist of people employed by the health authorities. There is yet another arm of support – voluntary organizations. A particularly good example of this is the hospice providing care for the terminally ill. Doctors and nurses working in this field, supported mainly by charity, develop a particular expertize and have teams that can visit patients in their own homes by arrangement with the general practitioner.

Other members of the health care team

Physiotherapists diagnose and treat patients' difficulties with movement, especially joints, and assist with rehabilitation after injury. Until recently they worked mainly in hospitals, but an increasing number now work in the community. GPs have direct access to their services.

Social workers can help many patients with problems in non-medical areas of their lives, e.g. living conditions, debts or problems with relationships or child care. The intervention of social workers at an early stage can often help in tackling patients' problems, although these may be closely related to medical conditions for which they consult their doctor. In some areas, GPs employ their own social worker because of the support he/she can give to patients who visit their doctor because they do not know where elso to go.

Counsellors may be employed by GPs or attend their surgeries for designated sessions; early intervention by a counsellor who has time to listen to patients' non-medical problems can help to avert a critical situation.

Dietitians and other care staff advise on the best food and drink for particular medical conditions. Some health centres and GP practices have a dietitian attending for designated sessions, working closely with members of the primary health care team.

Occupational therapists help patients to resume a normal life after mental or physical illness through activity-based treatments, and the provision of aids to living. They will also assess what alterations are needed to enable elderly or disabled people to continue living at home.

Speech and language therapists help patients who have communication difficulties, especially after stroke or injury. They are trained to diagnose and treat all forms of speech disabilities, disorders of language and articulation in children.

Chiropodists play an important part in helping the elderly, who frequently have debilitating toe and foot problems, to maintain an active role in the community.

Audiometricians do much in helping those with hearing disabilities to live a normal and active life.

Other specialist nurses

Specialist nurses working in the community also include:

- school nurse
- stoma care nurse
- paediatric nurse
- geriatric nurse
- local authority clinic nurse.

Health promotion

Approximately 20 years ago, health education was a new field seeking to make information about health matters available to anyone who wanted it. Health education councils generated literature, visited surgeries, schools and hospitals, to circulate information. In the last five years there has been an increase in health promotion in doctors' surgeries which has supplemented health education. Every opportunity is taken to draw attention to health issues, advise individuals to bring them to a point of decision to make changes in their lifestyle and then give out literature to further educate on how and why to make changes. Health promotion draws attention to the need to change, and educates sufficiently to enable a patient to make an informed choice to change. Support during the change process and further education with literature must then follow. The terms 'education' and 'promotion' refer to different aspects, but to effect change in patient behaviour the two must work hand in hand.

General practitioners and health care providers have been required to extend their services into promotion of health, as well as looking after the sick. Surgeries have implemented health promotion clinics, such as well-man and well-woman, where patients are asked details of their lifestyle and give advice on how they might prevent ill-health by changes to diet, drinking habits, smoking, exercise and so on. Where needs such as help in giving up smoking are identified, specific clinics are then provided in some surgeries, so that patients benefit from peer group support.

However, all the primary health care team, including receptionists and secretaries, are now required to be far more aware of promoting health. Just as one would find it difficult to accept advice from an obviously overweight practice nurse advising that one must lose at least two stones in weight in the next six months, it is important that health care staff present a healthy image – which may include not being seen smoking – to back up the message that the practitioners and other health professionals give out daily.

Patient waiting areas should be used to the full to promote health, with good quality notices tidily pinned up on notice boards, and to educate by leaflets available for patients to read whilst waiting or to take home. It may be the practice nurse's responsibility to maintain notice boards and supplies of leaflets, but it is important that receptionists keep their eyes open and draw the nurse's attention to notice boards that are looking unkempt or leaflet supplies that are running low.

General practices have also found that 'open days' are an excellent opportunity to give out health promotion messages, when patients are invited into the surgery perhaps on a Saturday afternoon to have blood pressure and cholesterol checks, and so on.

The educational aspect is supported in most schools who ask health visitors and social workers to speak to children and answer questions about what they can do to help themselves. Schools may also invite specific organizations, such as ASH (anti-smoking) or local AIDS charities to educate students about their particular area of expertize.

Since there are 1001 sources of educational information the role of staff is to be aware of where materials can be obtained for a wide range of subjects, so that literature can be obtained without undue delay. Where literature is not free, details of costs might be kept on record along with the addresses and contact numbers.

The government is making funding available for health promotion in surgeries by paying doctors who achieve targets for health promotion, but it is very difficult to audit the results. The range of effects on individual lives that might contribute to ill health makes it impossible to generalize about how effective any one particular message might have been. However, research to date shows that eating 'healthily', regular exercise and moderation in alcohol intake, along with refraining from smoking, all contribute to remaining healthier for longer. Where large scale health promotion in partnership with health education has been government sponsored, as in Finland, treatment for and deaths from heart disease have been reduced.

Therefore, it is part of the role of the receptionist to support initiatives to promote better health, not only by being aware of the advice given out by doctors and health professionals, but advising patients to attend health promotion clinics or events put on by the surgery, and by themselves presenting a healthy image to patients.

Local authority social services

Major local authorities have a social services committee, with an appointed director in charge of its social services department, who co-ordinates and administers the authority's social services.

Secretaries and receptionists inevitably will be asked by patients for information and advice about social services provision, and should be in a position of having the relevant information readily available to deal with such queries in a helpful, positive way.

Structure and social services provided

Figure 12.1 demonstrates the structure of a typical social services department. The organization of the department will vary from area to area, but there are usually at least five main sections of a social services department:

- residential services
- field work services
- provision of training facilities
- hospital social work
- administration.

The following is a summary of services provided by social services committees:

- *Care of the elderly* – This includes both field work services carried out within the community and residential care.
- *Care of the physically handicapped* – Blind, deaf, dumb, hearing difficulties, spastic, epileptic, paraplegics and other disabled persons.
- *Social work advice to the homeless* – Provision of permanent accommodation, care of homeless families, advice and help on prevention of homelessness, bed and breakfast accommodation.

Note: Those who are homeless are 'priority'. 'Priority' means anyone who has one or more children living with them; anyone who is made homeless, e.g. fire or flood; any household which includes one or more people who are elderly or mentally/physically handicapped, or suffer from physical disability; battered wifes; pregnant women. The homeless are also divided into those made *homeless by chance* and those made *homeless intentionally*.

- *Child care services* – Child care protection/supervision; acceptance of parental responsibility for children committed into care of the local authority; control of residential units; admission units; reception centres; residential nurseries; children's homes; community homes

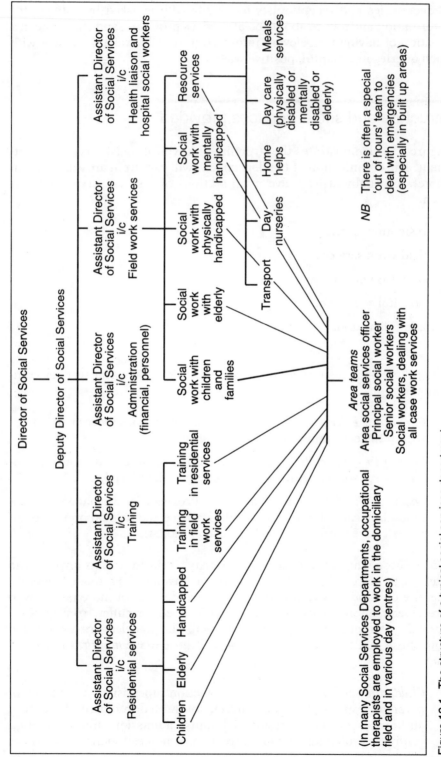

Figure 12.1 The structure of a typical social services department.

with education on the premises and classifying homes; adoption services; child abuse/prevention of child abuse services.

- *Social work and family case work dealing with mental disorder* – Provision of social workers; adult training centres; workshops; residential accommodation (hostels).

- *Day care for children under five years of age* – Provision of day nurseries, supervision of private nurseries and childminders.

- *Provision of home carers* – (See page 200).

- *Care of unsupported mothers* – Including residential care.

- *Hospital social workers* – Provision of social work services for hospital patients.

- *Work in the field of alcohol and drug abuse.*

Social work teams

A team of area social workers undertake all the case work for family and clients, so that problems can be considered as a whole, thus leading to family social services, helping all kinds of social problems in the family. Teams are made up of specialist social workers, for example, specialists in child care, mental illness or handicap, physical handicap and in the care of the elderly. It is the area social work team which usually co-ordinates the allocation of:

- home carers
- meals on wheels
- day nursery places
- vacancies in residential homes for the elderly
- residential accommodation for children.

Health and social services liaison

Social services work in close liaison with the local health authority to provide support and help in the community to patients recently discharged from hospital, or are suffering from a disabling condition. The necessary adaptations, gadgets and aids for these people that are vital for their rehabilitation are supplied by the occupational therapy section of the social services department.

A community physician, who is a specialist in community medicine, is responsible for liaison between health and social services. Social workers now visit medical practices and health centres, where they meet general practitioners, health visitors, community nurses and school nurses working from these centres.

Community care

Social services departments will continue to work closely with health authorities to plan and provide 'care packages' to give the support people need to help in their daily lives, and may be available from local government and health authorities. It involves both social and health care and the government will continue to encourage purchasers and providers to work with local authority partners to ensure that arrangements for community care work effectively. One of the major aims of community care is to enable people to maximize their independence by living in their own home for as long as possible, and when this is no longer practicable, to find them a homelike place to live.

Summary

The foregoing is intended to stress the importance to secretaries and receptionists of having sources of information at their finger-tips so that they are able to answer, with knowledge and understanding, the numerous and diverse questions put to them by patients and their relatives.

13

Training and development

Training and development should also be considered as ways of improving your personal effectiveness. Before we consider this in more detail, it is important to distinguish between:

- training
- education
- development.

Training is a systematic process for developing the skills, knowledge and attitudes, applied to a specific type of work. It is the process of bringing a person to an agreed standard of competence by practice or instruction.

Education is the process of acquiring background knowledge and skills. It does not have to be specific to a particular area of work.

Development is a course of action which enables individuals to realize their potential for growth and promotion in an organization.

Well-trained receptionists and secretaries are valued members of the work team, and are better able to understand, value and contribute to the smooth running of the medical practice or hospital department.

Excellent training courses are available and may be provided as in-house training taking place in the work environment, or by external training providers, for example, health authorities and colleges of further education (see Appendix 3). Training courses leading to a recognized qualification may necessitate attendance at a college on a day release basis, or may be provided as short training courses taking place in the evening.

National vocational qualifications (NVQs)

More and more training and development programmes and learning materials are designed to provide the underpinning knowledge and understanding which facilitates the achievement of competence towards NVQs.

NVQs are based on what people need to be able to do to carry out their jobs competently – they are work-based competences, which are assessed in the workplace. The qualifications are based on completion of units and elements and achievement of stated standards of performance criteria.

NVQs are assessed on the production of evidence of achievement, and secretaries and receptionists wishing to achieve NVQs should gather evidence in the form of a 'portfolio'. A portfolio is a collection of evidence demonstrating competence which can be based on previous as well as current learning.

Career structure

Secretaries and receptionists working in the field of health care are in a position, with their experience and further training, to progress to achieve the position of senior secretary or receptionist, and could well be considered sufficiently competent to progress further to a supervisory or management role within the organization.

An opportunity to discuss career development and any training needs could be identified at your annual performance appraisal, and a personal development plan arranged.

Summary

Training and development contribute to developing your personal effectiveness as a medical secretary or receptionist, and also to being a more effective, highly valued member of the work team.

There are several professional organizations and associations offering recognized qualifications. Your practice manager, training manager or your local college will be able to provide you with further information.

Further reading and reference books

Medical secretaries and receptionists should know the sources from which information can be obtained. The following list will be of value.

Medical reference

- *Medical Dictionary – Dorland's Pocket Medical Dictionary*
  Pocket Medical Dictionary, Churchill Livingstone.

- *The Medical Directory* – Consists of two volumes containing a directory of all qualified medical practitioners with addresses, qualifications and posts held. Information about hospitals is also included. There will usually be a recent copy at your place of employment.

- *First Aid Manual* – The authorized manual of St John's Ambulance Association, St Andrew's Ambulance Association and the British Red Cross Society.

- *British National Formulary* – This contains accurate information about all proprietary drugs.

- *MIMS* – A monthly publication listing all proprietary drugs and their uses.

General reference

English

- *The Concise Oxford Dictionary* or *Chambers Dictionary*

- Fowler's *Modern English Usage* – A helpful reference book for problems relating to English usage and grammar.

- Roget's *Thesaurus of English Words and Phrases* – This book lists words according to their meaning.

Information about correct forms of address will assist the secretary in ascertaining decorations, honours and qualifications, and placing them in the correct sequence. For example:

- Black's *Titles and Forms of Address*
- Debrett's *Peerage and Baronetage*
- *Who's Who*.

Travel information/guides

The secretary may find the following helpful, but up-to-date information should always be obtained from appropriate sources:

- Railway and Airways Guides
- Railway timetables
- Automobile Association (AA) and Royal Automobile Club (RAC) – These handbooks given useful information for motorists and details of hotels, etc.

Addresses and telephone numbers

Reference can be made to telephone directories and *Yellow Pages* for addresses and telephone numbers and listings of names under professions or trades.

The Post Office Directory can be used for detailed information of streets and occupiers of each house/shop etc.

General

- *Whitaker's Almanac*
- *Guide to your Local Social Services Provision*
- *Post Office Guide*
- *Voluntary Services Guide*
- *Pear's Cyclopaedia*.

Further reading

Allan D and Quinlan C (1995) *Making Sense of Computers in General Practice*, Radcliffe Medical Press, Oxford.
Ellis N (1994) *Making Sense of General Practice*, Radcliffe Medical Press, Oxford.

Ellis N and Chisholm J (1994) *Making Sense of The Red Book*, 2nd edn, Radcliffe Medical Press, Oxford.

Robbins M and Wetherfield J (1994) *Terminology for Medical Administrators*, Radcliffe Medical Press, Oxford. This book contains useful terminology for medical administrators.

Harding H (1990) *Secretarial Procedures: Theory and Application*, 2nd edn, Pitman Publishing, London.

Harrison J (1993) *Practical Office Procedures*, 3rd edn, Pitman Publishing, London.

Hippocratic Oath

I solemnly pledge myself to consecrate my life to the service of humanity.

I will give to my teachers the respect and gratitude which is their due;

I will practise my profession with dignity;

The health of my patient will be my first consideration;

I will respect the secrets which are confided in me, even after the patient has died;

I will maintain by all the means of my power, the honour and the noble traditions of the medical profession;

My colleagues will be my brothers;

I will not permit considerations of religion, nationality, race, party politics or social standing to intervene between me and my patients;

I will maintain the utmost respect for human life from the time of conception; even under threat I will not use my medical knowledge contrary to the laws of humanity; I make these promises solemnly, freely and upon my honour.

Training programmes

The following are a selection of the principal nationally validated training programmes.

Practice Receptionist Programmes 1, 2 and 3

PRP training programmes can be used to provide knowledge evidence towards Administration, NVQ Level 2 qualifications through RSA Examination Boards.

Hospital Receptionist Programmes, 1 and 2

Certificate of Attendance issued on behalf of National Association of Health Authorities and Trusts

Radcliffe Medical Press Ltd
18 Marcham Road
Abingdon
Oxon OX14 1AA
Tel: 01235 528820

Association of Medical Secretaries, Practice Adminstrators and Receptionists (AMSPAR)

AMSPAR
Tavistock House North
Tavistock Square
London WC1H 9LN
Tel: 0171 387 6005

Diploma in Medical Reception
Diploma in Medical Secretarial Duties
Diploma in Practice Management

RSA Examinations Board – Medical Audio-Typing
Medical Shorthand
Medical Word Processing

Examinations and certificates at different levels

RSA Examinations Board
Westwood House
Westwood Way
Coventry
Warks CV4 8HS
Tel: 01203 470033

Medical terminology

Some components of words referring to body structures

A knowledge of these words will help you to deduce the meanings of many of the medical terms you hear and see in the course of your work.

Word	Pertaining to
aden	gland
angi	vessels (esp. blood vessels)
arthr	joint(s)
aur	ear(s)
cardi	heart
caud	tail
cephal	head
cheil	lip(s)
chole	biliary system
cholecyst	gall-bladder
chondr	cartilage
col	colon
cyst	bladder
derm	skin
enter	intestine
fibr	fibrous tissue
gastr	stomach
gloss	tongue
haem or aem	blood
hepat	liver
hyster	uterus
labi	lips
lymph	lymphatic system
mamm, mast	breast(s)
myel	bone marrow or spinal cord
myo	muscle(s)
nephr	kidney(s)
ocul, ophthal	eye
onych	nails
orch, orchid	testes
or	mouth

os, oste	bone(s)
ot	ear(s)
pneumon	lung(s)
proct	rectum
pyel	kidney pelvis
ren	kidneys
rhin	nose
salping	uterine tubes
sial	salivary glands
spondyl	vertebra(ae)

Suffixes

Suffix	Meaning	Term	Definition
-algia	pain	arthralgia	joint pain
-ac)	pertaining	cardiac	pertaining to the heart
-al)	to		
-ar(ary)		vascular	relating to the circulatory system
-ic)	referring		
-ory)	to		
-ous	denoting	cutaneous	pertaining to the skin
-aemia	blood	hyperglycaemia	high blood sugar
-cele	swelling	cystocele	hernia of the bladder
	hernia	myelocele	protrusion of spinal cord through vertebrae
-centesis	puncture	paracentesis	puncture of a cavity
		thoracocentesis	aspiration of pleural cavity
-cyte	cell	leucocyte	white blood cell
-desis	binding fixation	arthodesis	surgical fixation of a joint
-dynia	pain	pleurodynia	pain in the inter-costal muscles
-ectasis	dilation	atelectasis	abnormal dilation of bronchus or bronchi
-ectomy	removal excision	tonsillectomy	removal of tonsils
-genic	origin	bronchogenic	originating in bronchi
-genesis	forming, producing	pathogenesis	producing disease
-gram	tracing, recording	venogram	recording (X-ray) of veins
-graphy	process of recording	arteriography	X-ray of arteries
-iasis	condition of, presence, formation of	lithiasis	formation of stones
		cholelithiasis	formation of stones in gall-bladder
-itis	inflammation	carditis	inflammation of heart

		rhinitis	inflammation of mucous membrane of nose
-logy	study of	cytology	study of cells
-malacia	softening	osteomalacia	softening of bone
-megaly	enlargement	cardiomegaly	enlargement of heart
-oid	like, resembling	osteoid	like bone
-oma	tumour	osteoma	tumour of bone
-osis	disease, abnormal condition	spondylosis	disease of spine
-pathy	disease	myelopathy	disease of spinal cord
-penia	lack of	leucopenia	deficiency of white blood cells
-phasis	ability to speak	dysphasia	difficulty in speaking
-phagia	ability to swallow	dysphagia	difficulty in swallowing
-phobia	fear of	agoraphobia	fear of open spaces
-pnoea	breath	dyspnoea	difficulty in breathing
-rrhage	a bursting out	haemorrhage	an escape of blood from the vessels
-stasis	arrest, or cessation, a halting	haemostasis	the arrest of a flow of blood
-trophy	nourishment	atrophy	to waste away
-uria	pertaining to urine	haematuria	presence of blood in urine

Prefix

Prefix	Meaning	Term	Definition
a-	absence, lack of	amnesia	loss of memory
ab-	from, away from	abduct	move away from mid-line of body
ad-	to, towards	adduct	move towards the mid-line of body
an-	absence, lack of	anaesthesia	loss of sensation
ante-	before	antepartum	before delivery
anti-	against	antiseptic	agent used against bacteria
brady-	slow	bradycardia	slow heart bear
contra-	opposite	contralateral	opposite side
circum-	around	cirumoral	around the mouth
com-	with	compound	to mix or fuse
con-	joined	congenital	present at birth
di-	disengage	diarthrosis	to separate from a joint
dia-	through, by means of		
ec-	out from	ectopic	not in normal place
endo	within	endometrium	lining of the uterus
exo-	outside	exogenous	produced outside

hypo-	beneath	hypotension	below normal blood pressure
infra-	under	infrapatellar	under the keecap
inter-	between	intercostal	between the ribs
intra-	within	intracellular	within a cell
mega-	large, abnormally enlarged	megacolon	abnormally large (dilated) colon
micro-	abnormally small	microscopic	visible only with aid of microscope
onc-	pertaining to tumours	oncology	scientific study of tumours
para-	near beside	paravertebral	beside the vertebra
peri-	around	pericardium	around the heart
pre-	forwards	prenatal	before birth
pro-	in front of	prognosis	forecast (of course of disease)
retro-	backwards	retroflexion	bending backward
sym-	beside	symphysis	growing together
syn-	along	synapse	joining of two neurons
tachy-	rapid	tachycardia	rapid heartbeat
trans-	across	transurethral	through the urethra

Some of the most commonly used abbreviations

AID	artificial insemination donor
AIDS	acquired immune deficiency syndrome
APH	antepartum haemorrhage
ASD	atrial septal defect
bd	twice per day
BI	bony injury
BP	blood pressure, British Pharmacopeia
CDH	congenital dislocation of the hip
CSF	cerebrospinal fluid
CNS	central nervous system
CT	computerized tomography
CAT	computerized axial tomography
CSU	catheter specimen of urine
CVP	central venous pressure
CVS	cardiovascular system
D&C	dilatation and curettage (uterine)
DLE	disseminated lupus erythematosus
DNA	did not attend (or deoxyribonucleic acid)
DS	disseminated sclerosis
DU	duodenal ulcer
D&V	diarrhoea and vomiting
DVT	deep vein thrombosis
DXRT	deep X-ray therapy

ECG	electrocardiography
EDD	expected date of delivery
ENT	ear, nose and throat
ESR	erythrocyte sedimentation rate
EUA	examination under anaesthetic
FB	foreign body
FHH	fetal heart heard
FDIU	fetal death in utero
GU	gastric ulcer
Hb	haemoglobin
HRT	hormone replacement therapy
IM	intramuscular
Ig	immunoglobulin
ISQ	in status quo (unchanged)
IUCD	intrauterine contraceptive device
IUD	intrauterine death or intrauterine (contraceptive) device
IV	intravenous
LB	loose body
MI	myocardial infarct
MRI	magnetic resonance imaging
MS	multiple sclerosis, mitral stenosis
MSU	midstream specimen of urine
NAD	no abnormality detected
NAI	non-accidental injury
NG	new growth
NYD	not yet diagnosed
OA	osteoarthritis
OT	occupational therapy
PET	positron emission tomography
PID	prolapsed intervertebral disc
PM	post morten
POP	plaster of Paris
PPH	post partum haemorrhage
PR	per (through) the rectum
PUO	pyrexia of unknown origin
PV	per (through) the vagina
RA	rheumatoid arthritis
RBC	red blood cell
RH	rhesus factor
SMR	submucous resection of nasal septum
SOB	shortness of breath
SOL	space-occupying lesion
SOS	if necessary
SPECT	single photon emission computer tomography
TB	tuberculosis or tubercle bacilli
tds	three times a day
THR	total hip replacement
TPR	temperature, pulse and respiration
Ts & As	tonsils and adenoids
TUR	transurethral resection (of prostate)
UTI	urinary tract infection
VD	venereal disease
VVs	varicose veins

WBC	white blood cells
WR	Wassermann reaction
XR	X-ray

Medical symbols

♀	male
♂	female
#	fracture
Δ	diagnosis
R_x	recipe (for prescription–"take thou")
+ve	positive
–ve	negative
c̄	with
s̄	without
1/7	one day
3/7	three days
1/52	one week
1/12	one month

Abbreviations used in prescribing

Abbreviation	Latin equivalent	English meaning
aa	ana	of each the amount
ac	ante cibum	before food
bd (or bid)	bis die (bis in die)	twice daily
c̄	cum	with
hn	hac nocte	tonight
mane	mane	in the morning
mdu	more dicta utendus	as previously directed
m et n	mane et nocte	morning and night
nocte	nocte	at night
om	omni mane	every morning
on	omni nocte	every night
pc	post cibum	after food
prn	pre re nata	whenever necessary
qds	quater die sumendum	four times a day
qid	quater in die	four times a day
sos	si opus sit	if necessary
stat	statim	immediately
td (or tid)	ter die (ter in die)	three times a day
tds	ter die sumendum	three times a day

Investigations

Digestive system

Test	Reason for test
Oral cytology	Detection of early cancer in the elderly
Oesophagoscopy (visual inspection of oesophagus)	Investigation of tumours, strictures Removal of foreign bodies
Gastroscopy (visual inspection of stomach)	Investigation of abnormalities, e.g. gastric ulcer, carcinoma
Liver function tests (LFTs)	Liver disease. Obstructive jaundice. Haemolytic jaundice
Endoscopic retrograde cholangio pancreatography (ERCP)	Detection of pancreatic cancer
Glucose tolerance tests (GTTs)	To test the patient's ability to stabilize his/her blood level
Laparoscopy (visual inspection of abdominal cavity)	Investigation of lower abdominal pain
Proctoscopy (visual inspection of anal canal and lower rectum)	Detection of haemorrhoids, or growths
Colonoscopy (visual inspection of colon)	Investigation of malignant changes or for biopsy
Sigmoidoscopy (visual inspection of sigmoid colon)	Detection of growths, ulcerative colitis
Examination of faeces	Diagnosis of gastric/duodenal ulcers/ carcinoma

Investigations and tests relating to haematology and blood transfusion

Test	Reason for test
Haemoglobin (Hb) estimation	Detection of abnormalities, e.g. poly- cythaemia, anaemia
Red cell count (RBC)	
Haematocrit or packed cell volume (PCV)	Routine blood investigations for presence of abnormalities
Mean corpuscular haemoglobin (MCH)	
Mean corpuscular haemoglobin concentration (MCHC)	
Erythrocyte sedimentation rate (ESR)	A test to screen for systematic disease (or progress of disease) e.g. inflammatory and autoimmune disease, malignancy, serious infection

White cell count (WBC)	Detection of disease and infection, e.g. pneumonia, leukaemia, appendicitis
Platelet count	Detection of disease, trauma, infection, inflammation, malignancy
Clotting time	To test extrinsic clotting system in diagnosis of haemophilia, obstructive jaundice, etc.
Prothrombin ratio	Investigation of haemorrhagic disorders, liver disease
Paul Bunnell	To diagnose infective mononucleosis (glandular fever)
Monospot	To diagnose infective mononucleosis (glandular fever)
Rose-Waaler (RA)	To diagnose rheumatoid arthritis
Latex fixation test	To diagnose rheumatoid arthritis
Antinuclear factor/antibody (ANF/ANA)	To diagnose systemic lupus erythematosus

Bacterial tests on blood

Widal reaction (WR)	Diagnosis of typhoid/paratyphoid and brucellosis
VDRL	Diagnosis of venereal disease
TPHA	Diagnosis of venereal disease
WR	Diagnosis of venereal disease
GCFT	Diagnosis of venereal disease
Guthrie's test	Estimation of blood level of phenylketonuria (PKU) in babies

---

Musculo–skeletal system

Disorders of bones and joints give rise to pain, deformity, swelling of bone and tissues, limitation of movement and secondary muscle wasting.

X-ray investigation is of value in diagnosis and assessment of response to treatment. Bone scanning is being increasingly used for detective of malignant conditions in bone.

Test	Reason for test
Arthroscopy (visual inspection of knee joint)	Diagnosis of disease/injury to interior of joint
Electromyography	Detection of muscular disorders, e.g. muscular dystrophy, myaestenia gravis and myotonia
Myelography	Detection of spinal lesions, e.g. tumours and prolapsed intervertebral disc
Radiculography	Similar procedure to myelography used to investigate the lumbosacral nerve roots

*(See also Miscellaneous investigations, page 234.)

Cardiovascular system

Test	Reason for test
Blood pressure (BP)	To detect disease Hypertension – abnormally high blood pressure Hypotension – abnormally low blood pressure
Angio-cardiography (injection of dye through catheter enabling X-ray of heart structure)	Detection of abnormalities of the heart and blood vessels
Electrocardiography (ECG) (recording of electrical activity of the heart)	To investigate heart disorders, e.g. coronary thrombosis, heart block
Echocardiography (EEG)	Diagnosis of valvular disease and pericardial effusion

Respiratory system

Test	Reason for test
Rhinoscopy (examination of interior of nose)	Removal of tissue for histology, or swab taken for bacteriology
Laryngoscopy	Examination of vocal cords, larynx and epiglottis, for growths and infections
Bronchoscopy (visual inspection of bronchi)	Diagnosis of growths. Tissue removal for biopsy
Sputum examination	Examination of sputum for blood, parasites, etc.
Pleural fluid	Detection of malignancy, chest injury, empyema, heart failure

Lung function tests

Test	Reason for test
Vital capacity of lungs (maximum amount of air which can be expired)	Measurement of amount of air expired by a patient. Diminished in lung disease
Wright's peak flow meter	Detection of lung disease

Nervous system

Test	Reason for test
Lumbar puncture	Examination of cerebrospinal fluid (CSF) and diagnosis of certain diseases of nervous system

Romberg's sign	Test for co-ordination. Used in diagnosis of multiple sclerosis, cerebral tumour, etc.
Kernig's sign	Diagnosis of meningitis, cerebral haemorrhage or meningism
Electroencephalogram (EEG)	Investigation of epileptic conditions and location of cerebral lesions
Electromyogram (EMG) (recording of electrical activity in a muscle)	Investigation of disease
Knee jerk	Detection of disease of nervous system

Pupil reflexes

Reaction to light	Detection of diseases of central nervous system

Eye tests

Optic discs	Detection of disease of central nervous system
Snellen's test	Measurement of extent of field of vision
Refraction tests	To correct defective vision by prescription of correct lens

Hearing tests

Audiometric tests	Determination of degree and type of hearing
Weber's test (tuning fork)	To distinguish between middle-ear and nerve deafness
Rinne's test	Detection of middle-ear deafness
Auriscopy (visual examination of middle ear)	Detection of infection and disease

Urinary system

Test	Reason for test
Routine Laboratory Examination	Detection of urinary infections, pyelonephritis. Haematuria (blood in urine)
Mid-stream specimen (MSU)	Nephritis, presence of parasites – tropical disease

Test for protein	Presence of protein in urine (albuminuria)
Test for sugar	Presence of sugar in urine (glycosuria)
Test for ketones	Presence of ketones in urine (ketonuria)
Test for blood	Presence of blood in urine (haematuria)

Renal efficiency tests

Blood urea	Impairment of renal function
Urea clearance test	To indicate extent of kidney damage
Cystoscopy (visual inspection of bladder)	Detection of disease of bladder. For biopsy of tissue/tumour
Intravenous pyelogram (IVP)	To test renal function. To demonstrate hydronephrosis, renal calculi, hydronephroma, etc.
Renal Biopsy	Specimen sent for histology

Pregnancy tests

Oestriol examination	Assessment of both placental and fetal function
Toxaemia of pregnancy	Urine tested for protein – to confirm condition
Amniocentesis	Estimation of fetal maturity. Detection of fetal defects, etc.
Cervical smear	Early diagnosis of cancer. Detection of infection and other conditions
Vaginal swab	To detect cause of vaginal discharge

Endocrine glands

Test	Reason for test
Thyroid function tests (TFTs)	Assessment of functioning of thyroid glands
Protein bound iodine (PBI)	Measurement of thyroid function

X-ray investigations

Test	Reason for test
Barium swallow	Detection of lesions of oesophagus. Demonstration of hiatus hernia
Barium meal	Detection of lesions of stomach and duodenum
Barium meal with follow-through	Detection of lesions of small and large intestines
Barium enema	Detection of disease and obstruction of the bowel
Double contrast radiography	Detection of small changes in gastric mucosa, e.g. early carcinoma
Cholecystography	To demonstrate presence of gall stones
Intravenous cholangiogram	To demonstrate bile duct obstruction from growth or stones
Arthrogram	To outline joint cavity
Bone scan	Detection of secondary tumours
Angiography	Demonstration of obstruction, aneurysm or abnormal course (of blood vessel)
Aortogram	Angiogram of aorta
Arteriogram	Angiogram of arteries
Venogram	Angiogram of veins
Bronchography	Diagnosis of bronchiectasis and other bronchial abnormalities
Lung scan	Demonstration of tumours
Mammography	Detection of early malignancy of breast
Myelogram	Examination of spinal cord for obstruction and other defects
Encephalogram	Detection of cerebral tumours
Ventriculogram	To confirm cerebral tumour

Skin tests

Mantoux test	Skin test for sensitivity to TB by dilute intradermal injection of tuberculin
Heaf test	Similar to Mantoux, but using multiple-puncture technique
Kveim test	Intradermal injection to diagnose sarcoidosis

Miscellaneous investigations

Radiography

X-rays are one of the most frequently requested investigations used by physicians. They are painless unless used in conjunction with a contrast media, which may cause discomfort; they are quick and easy to perform, but may be frightening for the patient.

X-rays are a form of electromagnetic energy of a short wavelength which have the ability to penetrate tissues.

Plain X-rays are commonly carried out on the chest, the abdomen, skull and limbs in order to study bones for bone disease, fractures, etc. Contrast media may be used to visualize soft tissues and organs.

Ultrasonography (ultrasound)

Ultrasound is a non-invasive diagnostic procedure used to view body structures. It is convenient, safe and a comparatively inexpensive investigation. It does not use ionizing radiation and is thus safer than radiography. Ultrasound examinations are carried out on the following structures:

- the brain – electroencephalography
- the arteries and veins
- the heart – echocardiography
- the kidney, liver and pelvis.

In obstetrics its main use is to demonstrate fetal size and growth, and the position of the placenta.

Computerized tomography

Computerized tomography (CT) scanning is an X-ray technique which uses a computer to reconstruct an image of a layer of tissue in the body. The CT scanner can image the three main cavities of the body (head, thorax and abdomen). It is mainly used for detecting lesions such as tumours and cysts in the body.

Nuclear magnetic resonance imaging (NMRI)

This form of investigation is now widely used in medicine, and is often referred to as MRI. It uses radio-frequency radiation in the presence of a magnetic field to produce anatomical sections of the human body.

It is a non-invasive technique, it does not use ionizing radiation, and it penetrates the body structures of the body. In contrast with CT scanning, MRI can provide images in any anatomical plane.

Radioisotope scanning

A radioactive isotope is an unstable isotope which decays or disintegrates, emitting radiation or energy. The energy source is inside the patient and is given either orally or intravenously.

Radioisotopic scans are performed to detect malfunction or abnormalities of bones, lungs, brain, heart, kidneys, gall-bladder, spleen and endocrine glands.

Thermography

This is a technique which measures and records heat energy from the skin surface. It is non-invasive and causes no discomfort. Films are taken in much the same way as a photograph is taken, and plates with these films are placed on the skin and changes of skin temperature are reflected on a colour map.

Thermography is mainly used to detect lesions of the breast, to evaluate drug therapy, to diagnose spinal root compression, and may be used to assess the progress of wound healing.

Tomography

This is a technique in which a single layer of tissue is examined. This is achieved by blurring the image of the tissues above and below the layer of tissue to be studied when the X-ray is taken.

Fluoroscopy

Fluoroscopy enables the function of organs to be directly visualized in motion on a flourescent screen, e.g. the heart beat, movement of the diaphragm and motility of the gastrointestinal tract can be observed and recorded.

Immunization schedules

Recommended immunizations for children

The schedule below is currently recommended by the Department of Health.

AGE	DISEASE	METHOD
At birth (high risk infants only)	tuberculosis hepatitis B	injection (BCG) injection
4 weeks (high risk infants only)	hepatitis B	injection
2 months	diphtheria, tetanus pertussis Haemophilus influenza type B (Hib) polio	one injection (DTP) injection by mouth (OPV)
3 months	diphtheria, tetanus pertussis Haemophilus influenza type B (Hib) polio	one injection injection by mouth (OPV)
4 months	diphtheria, tetanus pertussis Haemophilus influenza type B (Hib) polio	one injection (DTP) injection by mouth (OPV)
12–15 months (usually 14)	measles, mumps, rubella	one injection (MMR)
4–5 years	diphtheria, tetanus polio	booster injection booster by mouth (OPV)
10–14 years (girls only)	rubella	one injection
13 years	tuberculosis	one injection (BCG)
15–19 years	polio	booster by mouth (OPV)
16–18 years (school leavers)	tetanus	one injection

Recommended immunizations for adults

DISEASE	FREQUENCY	METHOD
Tetanus toxoid	booster every 10 years	one injection, or 3 at monthly intervals for those previously unvaccinated
Polio	booster every 10 years until age 40	by mouth (OPV)
For at-risk groups		
Influenza	annually (especially for the elderly)	injection
Hepatitis B	booster every 3 – 5 years	injections (in first instance, 3 over 6 months, followed by blood test)

Vaccinations for foreign travel

Travellers to hot climates and developing countries should be given immunizations and anti-malarial advice according to up-to-date recommendations which can be found in the *Pulse* and *MIMS* charts published monthly, and the patient's previous immunization status.

Incubation periods of some infectious diseases

The incubation period is the interval between the time of primary infection or contact with an infected person, and the appearance of the disease. The following information is a guide only as in some instances some of the diseases have been found to have an incubation period outside that of the stated range.

DISEASE OR CAUSATIVE ORGANISM	INCUBATION PERIOD
Amoebic dysentery	1–4 weeks
Bacillus cereus enteritis	1–5 hours
Botulism	2 hours – 8 days (usually 12–36 hours)
Brucellosis	1–8 weeks (usually 2–3 weeks)
Campylobacter enteritis	1–11 days (usually 2–5 days)
Chickenpox	10–21 days (usually 14–15 days)
Cholera	2–48 hours
Dysentery	1–7 days (usually 1–3 days)
German measles (rubella)	14–21 days
Infective jaundice (hepatitis A)	14–42 days
Hepatitis B	42 days – 6 months
Lassa fever	3–17 days
Legionnaire's disease	2–10 days
Leptospirosis	4–19 days (usually 7–12 days)
Malaria	8–25 days
Measles	7–21 days (usually 10–14 days)
Mumps	12–28 days (usually 16–18 days)
Polio	10–15 days
Rabies	2 weeks–5 years (usually 20–90 days)
Salmonella enteritis	6–72 hours
Scarlet fever	2–5 days
Typhoid fever	7–21 days
Whooping cough	5–21 days
Yellow fever	3–6 days

Abbreviations of qualifying degrees and further qualifications

BAO	Bachelor of the Art of Obstetrics
BC, BCh, BChir	Bachelor of Surgery
BM	Bachelor of Medicine
BS, ChB, CChir	Bachelor of Surgery
Bsc	Bachelor of Science
CCDC	Consultant in Communicable Disease Control
CM ChM	Master of Surgery
CPH	Certificate in Public Health
DA	Diploma in Anaesthetics
DCH	Diploma in Child Health
DCh	Doctor of Surgery
DCP	Diploma in Clinical Pathology
DDS	Doctor of Dental Surgery
DHyg	Doctor of Hygiene
DIH	Diploma in Industrial Health
DLO	Diploma in Laryngology and Otology
Dip Med Rehab	Diploma in Medical Rehabilitation
DM	Doctor of Medicine
DMR	Diploma in Medical Radiology
DO	Diploma in Ophthalmology
DObstRCOG	Diploma in Obstetrics of the Royal College of Obstetricians and Gynaecologists
DOMS	Diploma in Ophthalmological Medicine and Surgery
DPH	Diploma in Public Health
DPM	Diploma in Psychological Medicine
DR	Diploma in Radiology
DSc	Doctor of Science
DTH	Diploma in Tropical Hygiene
DTM	Diploma in Tropical Medicine
FDS	Fellow of Dental Surgery
FFA	Fellow of the Faculty of Anaesthetists
FFHom	Fellow of Faculty of Homeopathy
FFR	Fellow of the Faculty of Radiologists
FRCGP	Fellow of the Royal College of General Practitioners

FRCOG	Fellow of the Royal College of Obstetricians and Gynaecologists
FRCP	Fellow of the Royal College of Physicians of London
FRCPE	Fellow of the Royal College of Physicians of Edinburgh (may also be written as FRCPEd, FRCPEdin)
FRCPS	Fellow of the Royal College of Physicians and Surgeons
FRCPath	Fellow of the Royal College of Pathologists
FRCPsych	Fellow of the Royal College of Psychiatrists
FRCS	Fellow of the Royal College of Surgeons of England
FRCSE	Fellow of the Royal College of Surgeons of Edinburgh
FRIPHH	Fellow of the Royal Institute of Public Health and Hygiene
FRS	Fellow of the Royal Society
HVCert	Health Visitors Certificate
LAH	Licentiate of Apothecaries Hall, Dublin
LDS	Licentiate in Dental Surgery
LM	Licentiate in Midwifery
LRCP	Licentiate of Royal College of Physicians
LSA	Licentiate of Society of Apothecaries
MAO	Master of the Art of Obstetrics
MB	Bachelor of Medicine
Mcc, MCh, MChir	Master of Surgery
MChD	Master of Dental Surgery
MChOrth	Master of Orthopaedic Surgery
MCPath	Member of College of Pathology
MCPS	Member of College of Physicians and Surgeons
MD	Doctor of Medicine
MDS	Master of Dental Surgery
MFCP	Member of Faculty of Community Physicians
MFHom	Member of Faculty of Homeopathy
MHyg	Master of Hygiene
MMSA	Master of Midwifery of Society of Apothecaries
MPH	Master of Public Health
MRCGP	Member of Royal College of General Practitioners
MRCOG	Member of Royal College of Obstetricians and Gynaecologists
MRCP	Member of Royal College of Physicians of London
MRCPath	Member of Royal College of Pathologists
MRCPsych	Member of Royal College of Psychiatrists
MRCS	Member of Royal College of Surgeons of England
MS	Master of Surgery
RGN	Registered General Nurse
SEN	State Enrolled Nurse
SRN	State Registered Nurse
SRP	State Registered Physiotherapist

Other medical abbreviations (including job titles, organizations and non-clinical terms)

AHCPA	Association of Health Centres and Practice Administrators
AMSPAR	Association of Medical Secretaries, Administrators and Receptionists
BAMM	Association of Medical Managers
BMA	British Medical Association
BMJ	British Medical Journal
BNF	British National Formulary
BP	British Pharmacopoeia
BPC	British Pharmaceutical Codex
BRCS	British Red Cross Society
CHC	Community Health Council
CMB	Central Midwives Board
CME	continuing medical education
CNO	Chief Nursing Officer
DDA	Dangerous Drugs Act
DHA	District Health Authority
DN	District Nurse
DoH	Department of Health
DSS	Department of Social Security
FHSA	Family Health Services Authority
FPA	Family Planning Association
GDP	General Dental Practitioner
GMC	General Medical Council
GMSC	General Medical Services Committee
GMP	General Medical Practitioner
HV	Health Visitor
IHSM	Institute of Health Services Management
IMA	Independent Medical Adviser
LMG	Local Medical Committee
MAAG	Medical Audit Advisory Group
MDU	Medical Defence Union
MIMS	Monthly Index of Medical Specialities
MPS	Medical Protection Society
MSW	Medical Social Worker
NAHAT	National Association of Health Authorities and Trusts
NBTS	National Blood Transfusion Service
NHS	National Health Service
OT	Occupational Therapist
PACT	Prescribing Analysis and Costs
PGEA	Postgraduate Educational Allowance
QALY	Quality Adjusted Life Year
RCGP	Royal College of General Practitioners
RCN	Royal College of Nursing
RHA	Regional Health Authority
SHO	Senior House Officer

SI	Systeme International (units)
TQM	Total Quality Management
UKCC	United Kingdom Council for Nursing Midwifery and Health Visiting
WHO	World Health Organization

Useful addresses

Association of Community Health Councils
362 Euston Road
London NW1
Tel: 0171 388 4874

Association of Health Centre and Practice Administrators (AHCPA)
c/o Royal College of General Practitioners
14 Princes Gate
London SW7 1PU
Tel: 0171 581 3232

Association of Medical Secretaries, Practice Administrators and Receptionists (AMSPAR)
Tavistock House North
Tavistock Square
London WC1H 9LN
Tel: 0171 387 6005

British Medical Association (BMA)
BMA House
Tavistock Square
London WC1H 9JP
Tel: 0171 387 4499

Department of Social Security (DSS)
Eileen House
Elephant and Castle
London SE1 6BY
Tel: 0171 703 6380

General Medical Council (GMC)
44 Hallam Street
London W1N 6AE
Tel: 0171 580 7642

Institute of Health Services Management (IHSM)
75 Portland Place
London W1N 4AN
Tel: 0171 580 5041

King's Fund Centre Library
126 Albert Street
London NW1 7NF
Tel: 0171 267 6111

King's Fund College
2 Palace Court
London W2 4HS
Tel: 0171 229 9361

Health Service Commissioner (Ombudsman) for England
Church House
Great Smith Street
London SW1P 3BW
Tel: 0171 276 2035 or 3000
(Investigates complaints about health authorities in England)

Health Services Commissioner for Scotland
2nd Floor
11 Melville Crescent
Edinburgh EH3 7LU
Tel: 0131 225 7465

Health Services Commissioner for Wales
4th Floor
Pearl Assurance House
Greyfriars Road
Cardiff CF1 3AG
Tel: 01222 394621

Hospital Consultants and Specialists Association
The Old Court House
London Road
Ascot
Berks SL5 7EN
Tel: 01344 25052

Medical Defence Union
3 Devonshire Place
London W1N 2EA
Tel: 0171 4486 6181

Medical Protection Society
50 Hallam Street
London W1N 6DE
Tel: 0171 637 0541

National Association of Health Authorities and Trusts (NAHAT)
Birmingham Research Park
Vincent Drive
Birmingham B15 2SQ
Tel: 0121 471 4444

NHS Training Division
St Bartholomew's Court
18 Christmas Street
Bristol BS11 5BT
Tel: 01272 291029

Royal College of General Practitioners
14 Princes Gate
Hyde Park
London SW7 1PU
Tel: 0171 581 3232

Royal College of Obstetricians and Gynaecologists
27 Sussex Place
Regents Park
London NW1 4RG
Tel: 0171 262 5425

Royal College of Nursing (UK)
Henrietta Place
London W1M 0AB
Tel: 0171 580 2646

Royal College of Pathologists
2 Carlton House Terrace
London SW1Y 5AF
Tel: 0171 930 5861

Royal College of Physicians
11 St Andrew's Place
London NW1 4LE
Tel: 0171 935 1174

Royal College of Physicians, Edinburgh
9 Queen Street
Edinburgh EH2 1JQ
Tel: 0131 225 7324

Royal College of Physicians and Surgeons of Glasgow
232–242 St Vincent Street
Glasgow G2 5RJ
Tel: 0141 221 6072

Royal College of Psychiatrists
17 Belgrave Square
London SW1X 8PG
Tel: 0171 235 2351

Royal College of Surgeons
Nicolson Street
Edinburgh EH8 9DW
Tel: 0131 556 6206

Royal College of Surgeons of England
35–43 Lincoln's Inn Fields
London WC2A 3PN
Tel: 0171 405 3474

Royal Society of Medicine
1 Wimpole Street
London W1M 8AE
Tel: 0171 408 2119

Index

Note: page references in *italics* indicate illustrations. There may also be text on these pages.